How to Make It as a Student Nurse

How to Make It as a Student Nurse

CLAIRE CARMICHAEL
Registered Nurse/Assistant Lecturer
Birmingham City University
Birmingham, UK

ANN-MARIE DODSON
Senior Lecturer
Birmingham City University
Birmingham, UK

ELSEVIER

© 2024, Elsevier Limited. All rights reserved.

No part of this publication may be reproduced or transmitted in any form or by any means, electronic or mechanical, including photocopying, recording, or any information storage and retrieval system, without permission in writing from the publisher. Details on how to seek permission, further information about the Publisher's permissions policies and our arrangements with organizations such as the Copyright Clearance Center and the Copyright Licensing Agency, can be found at our website: www.elsevier.com/permissions

This book and the individual contributions contained in it are protected under copyright by the Publisher (other than as may be noted herein).

Notices

Practitioners and researchers must always rely on their own experience and knowledge in evaluating and using any information, methods, compounds or experiments described herein. Because of rapid advances in the medical sciences, in particular, independent verification of diagnoses and drug dosages should be made. To the fullest extent of the law, no responsibility is assumed by Elsevier, authors, editors or contributors for any injury and/or damage to persons or property as a matter of products liability, negligence or otherwise, or from any use or operation of any methods, products, instructions, or ideas contained in the material herein.

ISBN: 978-0-323-93190-8

Content Strategist: Andrae Akeh
Content Project Manager: Subodh Kumar
Cover Designer: Bridget Hoette
Marketing Manager: Deborah Watkins

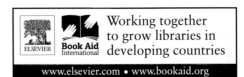

Working together
to grow libraries in
developing countries

www.elsevier.com • www.bookaid.org

Printed in the UK by Bell & Bain Ltd

Last digit is the print number: 9 8 7 6 5 4 3 2 1

This book is dedicated to all the amazing role models I have had in my life: the girl who couldn't boil an egg, my friend who said 'I can see you as a nurse', to all the residents I cared for who said 'you should be a nurse because you have such caring, gentle hands', my mentors as a student nurse, the amazing lecturers at Birmingham City University (City South Campus) who paved the way for me and to the lead nurses out there who are showing great leadership in nursing. This is also dedicated to every single student nurse right now – struggling and wondering how they will make it. You WILL make it, and you ARE amazing. Keep going! Never give up on your dreams. This is also dedicated to my parents, who passed away… I wish you could see me now and all I have achieved. Thank you for everything you taught me in life – the good, the bad and the ugly.

This book is based on my own experiences, opinions and advice from my own journey through nursing. Different universities and countries may differ from what I have experienced so far. Always check with your university or healthcare placement/trusts guidelines, policies and procedures before taking on any advice from others. Your journey into and throughout nursing is yours, so sit back and enjoy the amazing ride.

Nursing can be tough, hard going and exhausting. You have probably heard all of the negative press about nursing and are wondering how you are going to cope? What's going to be expected of you? What's placement like? What are the exams and assignments like? Don't panic! I'm here to help you along, wherever I can. You got this!

I am here to give you my personal lived experiences through my own nursing journey to help you, because that's what nursing is about: teamwork, collaboration and motivating each other to do this so that we can provide the best care possible for our patients.

In this book, I share my top tips, from applying to university to assignments, revision/exam preparation and placements. I hope it helps the future of our student nurses out there! Good luck! ☺

Disclaimer This book is to give you some personal tips and advice to help you. Only YOU can pass your degree.

CONTRIBUTORS

Dawn Jones
University of Dundee
Scotland, UK

Felicia Ikonmwosa
Birmingham City University
Birmingham, UK

George J. Blake
Residential Support Worker
Birmingham, UK

Mish Robinson
Birmingham City University
Birmingham, UK

Sez Francis
Chickenshed Theatre Company
Hertfordshire, UK

Stephen Wanless
Birmingham City University
Birmingham, UK

CONTENTS

CONTENTS

CHAPTER 1

Introductions

Hello, my name is… and this is my story so far.

Hello, my name is Claire Carmichael, and my pronouns are she/her.

As I start writing this book, I am 35 years old and currently living in Birmingham, UK. I have just started my third and final year of nursing and this has been a very long 10+-years journey for me. Spoiler alert – I am now 38 and a qualified nurse. I started writing this book in my second year of nursing and have been working on it slowly, piece by piece.

Let's get personal and let me start at the beginning – I am rewinding time back to my 7-year-old self. I grew up with my grandparents from the age of 2 years old when they became my legal guardians. I was 7 years old when my grandad was diagnosed with cancer, and he chose to die at home with us. He was a very stubborn man from what I can remember and that's exactly why he refused to go to hospital. This is potentially where I get my stubbornness from too. So, we had the district nurses come out and care for him at home and this was the first time I remember falling in love with nursing. I remember admiring these wonder women and how they behaved with my grandad; they showed care and compassion. However, I never realised nursing was my path until later in life.

I grew up caring for sick animals, mainly pigeons with broken wings; I would find them on the street and take them back to my nan and she would go a little bit mad at me for doing so. But I just wanted to help them, I can't bear to see anything suffer. I also used to make medicine and bandages from dock leaves, grass, vines and rose petals in the garden to use on my friends when they hurt themselves – luckily, they healed, and I didn't cause sepsis. So, what *did* I want to be growing up? I don't ever remember thinking about what I would be when I grew up. But I always remember having a little post office set and I loved sitting and stamping everything – I still love stamping things. So, I assume that I wanted to be some sort of professional stamper maybe.

Fast forward to my 16-year-old self. My nan had now passed away (cancer again!), and I was back living with my mother, which wasn't the best, but that's a whole different story. I had just got my GSCE results and had no idea where I wanted to go next. We don't all know where we want to go in life as soon as we leave school and even though I fell in love with nurses at

7 years old, I still didn't think about nursing as a career choice. I didn't think nursing was a role you could go into without having a professional family background etc. I saw nursing as such a high profession that someone like me could never be in. Furthermore, I didn't do well in my GSCEs: mostly D's and E's! This made me feel unconfident in my own abilities and that I was not worth enough to do anything great in my life. It didn't help that a kid at school said to me 'you'll be out on the streets selling the big issue!' So, I left school, and decided I would follow in my mother's footsteps and go and work at a hotel she worked at. I worked in hospitality for a few years, a mixture of housekeeping, reception and waitressing but it wasn't for me; I didn't feel like I had a purpose in life. Although housekeeping was one of my favourite jobs, I needed more in my life.

In 2005, I decided I needed a change and after a conversation with a friend, I applied for a care assistant job in a care home for the elderly. This is where I found my *real* love for nursing! I realised I genuinely cared about people and loved being the person who helped them live as full of a life as possible. It is also where I found my voice in protecting patients as I had to report a carer for the way she had been treating patients. Despite my realisation, I STILL had it in my mind that *I* couldn't be a nurse; I wasn't smart enough. My confidence was low, my self-esteem was on the floor and my grades were so poor I'd be laughed at by any professional (or so I thought). And then enter a young healthcare assistant, who I became good friends with for a while as well as a work colleague. During one mealtime, a patient asked for a boiled egg on toast. I watched her squirm and then she came and said to me quietly 'I've no idea how to boil an egg can you do this?' Haha. No disrespect or offence to anyone who can't boil an egg, but this made me laugh so much. I'd been cooking for myself since I was 16 years old, so this blew my mind a little bit. I think we were both 19/20 years old at this point. Anyway, she had told me she was going to be a nurse, she had confirmation and would start the diploma course in September. *THIS* is when I realised, 'If she can do it so can I! She can't even boil an egg!' (Again, no offence to anyone.) She was an amazing carer and so lovely. With her inspiration, I went out and got my NVQ level 2 and 3 in health and social care, alongside my numeracy and literacy certificates – which is all you needed to get into the nursing diploma back then. But when I went to apply for my nursing diploma, they *JUST* scrapped the diplomas and turned nursing into a degree-only profession. Which put me off a little bit again as I had heard of the 10,000-word dissertation and thought 'there is no way I could do that, I'm not smart enough!' But nursing is all I was good at and something I have always been confident in is my work. I know I do a fantastic job caring for others; I practice safely and practically. I have common sense which really goes a long way as well as working on my own initiative. I CAN DO THIS!

So, I then went off and did my access course (which is the equivalent of A-levels to get me onto a degree at university) and started my nursing degree in October 2012. Unfortunately, after a few months, I had to withdraw from the university and leave nursing. I won't go into too much detail as I don't want to break confidentiality. However, I will say, I was pretty much made homeless, with no money and nowhere to go by someone I had classed as a very good friend of mine. I had to move back in with my mother who lived in Milton Keynes at the time, and she was in the middle of moving to Suffolk! I tried to commute from Milton Keynes to Birmingham for placement whilst I tried to find somewhere to live, and I failed. My funds ran out eventually and so did my motivation. I felt powerless to go on and had no option but to leave. I took a couple of years out to work, get some money behind me, find somewhere to live and sort my life out.

I found the perfect job in March 2014 in sexual health and family planning services across Birmingham and Solihull as a healthcare assistant. I had been watching all the TV shows about 'the sex clinic' and really wanted to work there. I moved in an instant; again, I had nowhere to live. Fortunately, there was staff accommodation at the time at the old Selly Oak Hospital. I can't say it was the best, but it was a roof over my head and with in my budget. The building itself used to be an old hospital, the rooms converted into the bedrooms, and you had to run down the corridor to the bathroom through the dark and quite possibly haunted halls. I did finally move out into a house share with the loveliest of people. It took me two further attempts to get back into university due to being awful at interviews. I wish they would just come and watch me work or something, somewhere where I feel confident. But during interviews my mind always goes blank, they could ask me if the sky was blue, and I would say 'I don't know' haha.

However, I managed to bag my place at university and had the most amazing experience throughout my 3 years. Along the way, I met some wonderful people and have made friends for life from it.

Fast forward to today, I am a newly qualified nurse, and I got a first-class honours degree – I got a first in my dissertation too! It's been a long-winded road, but this means so much more to me because of my journey here. My advice to anyone out there, never give up on your dreams, no matter how long it takes you because that time is going to pass you by either way. Get up and do it now. Go, go, go! This degree has changed me so much so far. My confidence is slowly going up, I feel I AM worth something and I CAN be a fantastic nurse when I qualify. All thanks to being able to boil an egg. Hands up who loves eggs?

I mentioned I met some wonderful people along the way. One of these people is the lovely Ann-Marie Dodson (Fig. 1.1) who I have co-authored with on this book. She is the most determined and hard-working person I know; this is her story:

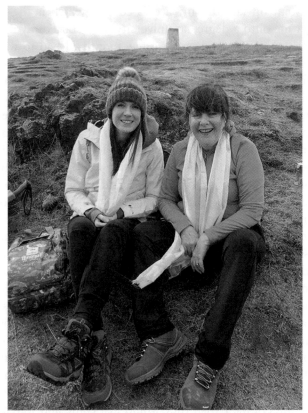

Fig. 1.1 Ann and Claire. (Claire Carmichael's personal Image.)

Ann-Marie Dodson

'I wanted to be a nurse from the age of four. As a severe asthmatic, I was considered a frail child. It changed my life journey as at a young age it was being planned to send me to Switzerland for the 'air', due to the gross pollution in Birmingham, where the death rates were very high in the winter smogs. I couldn't go to the Convent on a scholarship with all my friends as the GP felt a local grammar school was far better for my health rather than travelling across the city on a bus. So, I passed the 11+ exam and had an academic education at a local grammar school which meant that I was expected to go off to university where I studied geography. After getting a holiday job in a local hospital for the elderly I found my niche. I was so happy and fulfilled, but my parents and my school felt it was a waste of a good education. It was several years before I took courage and disobeyed them by getting a place on a nursing course after several failed attempts, as the nursing schools felt I was too qualified and would not be able to adapt to the very disciplined life as a student nurse in the 1970s. I got married and had a baby during my training which was frowned upon and caused conflict. However, nursing was my dream and I have never regretted a moment of it. I have been able to use my love of the outdoors and combine that with my career as a nurse. The skills that I acquired have not only been useful in my work setting but were used on occasion in emergency situations with my late father and husband. Nursing is such a privilege. You never stop learning about yourself, the work and the patients and families themselves. Such an immensely rewarding and satisfying career, one I would highly recommend but it does require hard work and commitment.'

Ann-Marie commenced her career in the NHS as a nursing auxiliary and qualified General Nurse in 1981 from Selly Oak School of Nursing where she worked in Medicine, Emergency Surgery and Intensive Care.

In 1989, she moved to the Queen Elizabeth hospital working in Renal, Liver and Intensive Care before qualifying as a clinical teacher and tutor to the intensive care course in 1993.

In 1995, she moved into higher education and ran a variety of critical care courses and worked as a programme director, apart from working on a variety of validations and projects, a notable one being taking students and staff in Nepal in 2013 on a study programme, whilst trekking to Everest base camp and Kala Patthar. She has also been an external examiner for a professional nursing body and a variety of universities.

CHAPTER 2

Applying to University: Personal Statement and Bagging that Interview

Here it is – you've made the brave, bold move to apply to university! The first thing you need to do is apply through UCAS. You can apply to up to five universities and there is a small fee of £25 for multiple choices and £20 for a single choice. (Correct as of September 2020 – UK-based only, fees and application process may change over time; double check this when you are applying.) Furthermore, applications open around May time to apply for the following year's programme at the university and the deadline is in October. So, you have a few months to apply. Make sure you have completed all steps on the UCAS application, including references, before hitting submit or it won't be accepted (UCAS, 2020a). Please check the UCAS website for all the information on applications and deadlines, as dates may vary between courses. However, I have also heard of students applying directly to one university. So, call the local universities you would like to go to and ask about their application process or check the university website for more details.

I also ask you to think about the university you want to go to. Which one? Where is it based? How do you choose which university to apply to? I didn't have any issues here, because I already had it in mind, I wanted Birmingham City University (BCU) and nowhere else. It was close to my home, easy access but I was also drawn to it. Like a moth to a flame, I fully believed that is where I was meant to be. To be honest, I know now it was where I was meant to be! Being at BCU gave me so many opportunities that I am not sure I would have had if I went anywhere else. I became the university's official vlogger, I started up the health section in the BCU magazine, and I became a high achievers recognition scheme scholar, which I haven't seen anywhere else. As a scholar, I was given funds of £2300 to go towards my personal development, which I fully used to get my online blog site going, to continue to vlog, I was able to buy a better laptop, camera and accessories with it! My personal development with this was a win–win situation really. It helped me gain more confidence, it gave me more opportunities to attend events and it all helped student nurses as well. Because just like this book, all of my blogs and vlogs were set up to help nurses out in any way I could.

I also became a 'buddy mentor' for international students which was THE best couple of weeks of my life. I signed up to help international students settle into university life and to Birmingham. During the 2 weeks I had to meet with a group of students, show them around the campus and then show them around Birmingham. I had a map of areas to show them, however, I took them to the best places I knew such as one of the best Indian street food restaurants I have ever been to. We had games and events. I ended up being a goalie during a football match at one point (haha) and I was ok! One of my best moments was when we did a treasure hunt around the university and my team won! So, we all gathered in the graduate plus office (it was tiny!) and there were loads of us, and I stood on the main desk to get a video of everyone in there – it was jammed packed – and we all chanted 'blue, blue, blue' (we were the blue team). I will never forget that moment, to be honest. However, my main reason for signing up was to help others, but this helped *me* grow. I discovered things about myself I never knew, it gave me confidence and I had the most fun ever if I'm honest. These are memories I will always keep with me, so remember this when you're looking around for a university, make sure it meets your needs.

When thinking about which university to attend, think about where your placements will be based as well. Because if you're on a 12-hour shift 7:00 a.m. to 19:00 p.m. you're going to want a shorter distance to travel. I was based on the other side of Birmingham and it took around 1.5 hours to get to some of my placements, which meant I had to leave home at around 5:00 a.m.! So please, bare this in mind when you are looking at a university. Make it easier for yourself if you can. Some of my top things to look for in a university to help you as a student nurse:

1. What support they have: Extra teaching sessions, any disability support, mental health support/counselling services if needed, library support, IT support.
2. Distance from your home for placements.
3. What facilities do they have: Library, personal development department, café/canteen, shop, computers etc.
4. What space do they have for you to learn: Dedicated learning spaces with computers, tables and seating.
5. Go to an open day and get a feel for the place and the staff there.
6. Visit university social media sites and see what students are saying about them.

So, if you have picked your university, or have a rough idea about where you want to go, now it's time to get the application in. But what should you write in your personal statement?

In your UCAS application you must write a personal statement. This can be up to 4000 characters (characters not words) long (UCAS, 2020b). I wanted to share with you how I structured my statement and the sorts of things I included. I really hope this helps you and I hope all the tips and advice make sense too. You can also ask friends and family to have a look at their statements to see what things they wrote and get an idea of how to write yours. But please, do not copy anyone else's statement as this is classed as plagiarism and you will not be accepted onto the course. Make your statement original and stand out.

Plagiarism: The practice of using or copying someone else's work or idea or work and pretending that you thought of it or created it

COLLINS DICTIONARY (2020)

I opened my personal statement with a quote from Mother Teresa. It was about looking after the ones you love from home. I felt this was appropriate for me, as I wanted to work in the community rather than the acute hospital sector. Putting a quote is always nice I think, as long as it is relevant to what you're writing, and you can link your statement to it. Again, it makes you stand out, but it's not really needed as such. I just personally thought it was a nice sentiment. These are all the top tips I used to write mine (Box 2.1).

BOX 2.1 ■ Top Tips for Writing Your Personal Statement

- Write it on word document first and then copy and paste when it's finalised and ready to submit.
- Talk about your skills, qualities and experience that you can bring to the course and why you're suitable for nursing.
- Avoid mentioning any of the university names in your statement as one statement does all universities – if you are using all five choices that is.
- Write about why you're applying for nursing and what interests you about this course.
- Your ambitions and career pathway.
- Mention any extracurricular activities you may take part in relevant to nursing/transferable skills.
- International students only – write about why you want to study in the UK. Your English language skills and any English courses or tests you've taken and why you want to study here in the UK rather than study in your own country.
- Mature students only – Mention all your experience and any courses you have recently done such as the access course.
- Write with passion, show your passion on the paper so they can see how much you want this.
- Try and stand out from the crowd! They will be reading hundreds of these personal statements, and you want to be remembered. Tell a funny story or put a nice quote in, something to make them remember you. I told a story about when I was younger and used to nurse injured pigeons at home and my nan would get so angry at me for it.
- Don't waffle or repeat yourself – I have read some personal statements, and people tend to say the same thing, just in a different way throughout their statement. Don't do that.
- Keep it relevant to nursing.
- Get someone to proofread your statement to check for grammar and spelling mistakes.

So, how I structured my statement was, I had my quote to start it off with then explained why I had added this quote. So, like I explained, I want to work within the community, then went on to explain why this was – so, my personal back story of having district nurses come to visit my grandad at home and watching them. I gave the story of 'nursing' injured pigeons to show my caring nature but to make them laugh too. This joined with the fact I had always worked within the community setting made me fall in love with this particular area of nursing. I then went on to discuss my skills relevant to nursing; if you have no experience in healthcare, you can still have transferable skills – communication, handling complex situations, team working, using your initiative etc., Bring these into the statement and how they can apply to nursing – sell yourself! Then I explained why I wanted to do the nursing degree (for me it was building that knowledge, gaining more skills to become a qualified nurse and give my patients the best care possible), I then went on to explain what I knew about the nursing degree: 50% theory and 50% practical (this may change in future), and how I would be completing many exams, assignments and placements to be assessed. Universities like to see you know what you are getting yourself into and the pressures you may face in nursing. I then brought it back to my skills, any extra activities I had done to prepare for the course and then where I saw my future as a qualified nurse and what it meant to me, bringing that passion and my goals into it. Think of your statement as an essay. You want an introduction, a main body and then your end/conclusion. Keep a good structure, keep it relevant, straight to the point, but shine!

Applying to University: Interview Tips

CONGRATULATIONS, YOU HAVE GOT AN INTERVIEW AT THE UNIVERSITY!

Trust me, I *know* how awful interviews can be. As I mentioned in the introduction, it took me two failed attempts to get into university. Please don't be disheartened if you get a 'no' this time around. I'm really glad I had that 'no' the first time around, because I wouldn't be where I am today if I had qualified any earlier. So, think of it as an opportunity rather than failing, you are not a failure! You either win in life or you learn; take this to learn and grow. Some tips if you aren't successful this time: ask for feedback on your interview so that you can improve next time, brush it off and try again – you *can* do this! All of my feedback from failed attempts in interviews was 'you didn't sell yourself enough'. And that one thing was the decision between me and another person. So please don't forget to sell yourself, because sometimes it's that small thing that decides between you and someone else getting that place. And you deserve this place as much as anyone else out there.

I remember my first-ever interview so well. I was nervous as ever and really wanted this so much. I had a Maths and English test first and if you passed this section, you then went on to get the interviews. We did this in groups initially and luckily, I passed. We then went into a small room to watch a video of a 'patient' and a 'healthcare worker'. We were to take notes throughout the video and write comments on what we thought were good care and poor care. Once we had watched the video, we were all called one by one into another smaller room for our interview. I had two people sat in front of me with clip boards of questions to ask me, and to be honest, they were very generic, normal questions. Nothing tricky as such, however, my mind went blank on one question in particular – name two of the 6 C's of Nursing and give examples of these. Could I think of a second one? No. My mind had gone blank because I was so nervous. I apologised and we moved on from the question. It was no wonder I had a rejection letter after that – the 6 C's of nursing and I couldn't remember! That was quite possibly one of the worst interviews I had ever done, but it gave me experience, and I was well prepared for the next time. And not only that, if I hadn't had got things so wrong in life, I wouldn't be here writing about it and helping others, so I am grateful for all these little things in life that knocked me back. So, please, take your time in your interview and try and remain calm to avoid this happening to you. Which I know is hard when you get so nervous, but the more you can practice before your interview and use breathing techniques to control your anxiety – hopefully, this will help you on the day.

What are the 6 C's of Nursing?

1. Care
2. Compassion
3. Communication
4. Commitment
5. Courage
6. Competence (NHS England, 2015)

I wanted to write a bit extra about the 6 C's of nursing and how important they are. It seems that some nurses may have lost their way, lost their motivation and love for the role of the nurse. With the tough times of staff shortages, cuts made to healthcare, pay cap and then covid hitting, I can see how easily this can be done. So, I wanted to talk about this and hopefully bring some passion and hope into people's hearts.

Care. This should be the key one people think of when we ask about the 6 C's – care. But what does that mean to people? It can mean a variety of things to each and every one of you. To me, care is exactly what it says on the tin. To physically, mentally, emotionally, holistically want to help someone else in need. There are many definitions of 'care':

Noun: 'The process of caring for someone or something and providing what they need for their health or protection.'

Verb: 'Feel concern or interest; attach importance to something'
OXFORD DICTIONARY (n.d.)

To me, this comes naturally, I am a genuinely caring person, probably too much! I have a lot of empathy for others. I can't do enough for the patients I look after. I do go above and beyond for patients, it's the one thing I know I am good at. Because it must be so tough being in hospital, without your loved ones, alone and feeling like utter rubbish. All you want is your own bed and a decent cup of tea (or any beverage of choice). The last thing you want on top of this is a nurse that is stressed and has not got time to CARE for you. A nurse should speak to you in a professional manner, to show they care and want to help you. Not a nurse that is huffing and puffing because you're not well and pressed your buzzer for another sick bowl. So, remember, you are that patient's nurse; you have just become their hope of getting back to good health and back to their family. Stay kind.

Compassion. Goes hand in hand with care. You have to show you have feelings towards that patient. To show you're human and can connect with your patient. Show feelings of sympathy for what they are going through right now. It doesn't matter what happened at home when your toaster blew up and set off the smoke alarm. It matters what that patient is thinking and feeling and how YOU can make them feel better at least. If your mind is at home still, this will distract you from your patient.

Competence. This is your ability to do your job. Are you up to date with your training? Have you been trained on that hoist you're about to use on Patient X? Are you confident enough to give that injection and know it's the correct dose? If you're unsure or uneasy about something don't do it. This is how mistakes are made and patient care is put at risk. You wouldn't rewire your electrics at home unless you were 100% confident and trained to do so, so why put your patient at risk? And let's be honest, if you haven't got the first two C's (care and compassion) you probably wouldn't care if your patient is at risk or not, you will just chance it. If that's the case, maybe find a different job where people's lives are not at risk. I can understand the pressure of staff shortages and how people feel they HAVE to do something because of this, but is it worth it? Get help, get trained, call the on-call doctor for advice, talk to your ward doctor for advice, the ward manager – anything that is going to help you in that situation you're unsure of. As student nurses, we must work with our mentors and not work outside of our competencies. Do not just do something because your mentor has told you to – who says they aren't wrong? Ask questions all the time, know why you are doing something and know you can do it before making a mistake. This isn't painted by numbers, this is a person's life that could be at risk if you get it wrong. Stay safe and within your limits. Protect your patient, always.

Communication. You must communicate with your patient. Poor communication is something I have seen in the past between healthcare staff and a patient. To be honest, these were very good nurses and healthcare assistants, I just feel that there isn't enough training on communication with individuals with various needs.

Story Time. I was assisting with a patient with dementia, they had warned me before I went into the room with them that he gets 'very aggressive' and 'lashes' out. So, I said I would come in and help distract him and talk to him whilst they assisted him with his personal hygiene care. I was surprised to find the way they communicated with this patient was VERY different to the previous patient they had just been to (Patient × who had capacity). There was a lack of communication, they did not explain to the patient properly what they were doing as they were doing it. So, in the patient's eyes, they were just being rolled about and soapy water was thrown at them. They just started undressing the patient and washing them without telling the patient as they were doing it. *This* is why the patient gets aggressive – they were terrified. It's bad enough that they are in a room they don't recognise, with people they don't know, now their dignity has just gone out the door with their clothing. So, I was then explaining to the patient as it was going on, what they were doing as they were doing it. I was calm, I talked to the patient in short simple sentences in a low gentle tone, and told them they were safe, that the nurse/HCA were just washing them 'just for a moment, if that's ok' which seemed to calm the patient down. The staff said the patient was much better and calmer this time around than before when they have been to him. They didn't have any scratches on them and no swear words (in the end). These were well trained, good staff. Fantastic staff. I was so shocked to see that they didn't know how to communicate properly with a patient with dementia. This is common, I think. People fear the unknown. I feel there needs to be A LOT more extra training for staff to communicate properly with these patients. In fact, communication in general within healthcare is so poor from what I have seen. The moral of the story is, listen and talk to your patient, ALWAYS. If they don't understand, find ways to communicate through picture cards, writing, drawing, getting an interpreter. Anything to help your patient understand you and you them. There is a very good quote:

'Most people do not listen to understand; they listen with the intent to reply.'
STEPHEN. R. COVEY

Courage. I found a great quote for this:

'Courage is not the absence of fear but rather the assessment that something else is more important than fear.'
FRANKLIN D. ROOSEVELT

We think of courage as being brave. But as a nurse, every day you have the courage – to face the pain, to face the sadness of sick patients you look after. Everyone is affected differently in every way and it's the courage that gets you over it. It's the courage that helps you go into that patient's room, knowing that patient may have passed away and you're the person to find them. The courage to talk to family members about the patient's condition (where acceptable). The courage to do something incredible even though you are scared. We all have our fears in life. But it's the courage that lets us face our fears and allows us to conquer them. You need the courage to be open and honest as a nurse, to admit your mistakes and reflect and learn from them. To have the courage to stand up and tell a doctor they have got it wrong. In some cases, YOU know your patient more than them; YOU know what's what. If in doubt, question it. Have the courage to be an advocate for that patient, always, because you may be the person who saves their life.

And for nurses that are struggling to get up in the morning and face another 12-hour shift on the ward, when it's short-staffed and feeling like you can't go on, you have the courage to get up and go. You put your nurse face on, and you do it. You face that day, and you conquer it like a boss. You do that because you know that without you, that day will be even worse, and your patients suffer as a result. Why do *you* do it though? Because you have the first two of the 6 C's above. You CARE and you have COMPASSION even though times are tough. You are that patient's saviour. You are the nurse we need to multiply, clone, and put in every healthcare setting. We need more courage like this. Thank you for being you.

Commitment. This links with the courage part. You have to be committed to the role. Those nurses as discussed above, the ones who go to work every day despite knowing it's going to be a hard day, have commitment. I feel like hope should be an added word here too. They have commitment because they hope that it's going to get better. That it's just a bad day and tomorrow is a fresh day. It is being dedicated to your role, your patients and your colleagues. Attending the training on your days off because you know you need it to provide the best care for your patients. Student nurses, you are committed to this degree. You knuckle down, revise, learn, grow, follow advice from mentors, lectures, attend your mandatory training and show up. Twelve-hour shifts are long, colleagues and patients slowly become your family. You see them more than your own family. It takes commitment to do that. We do this because we want to be that nurse as above. We want to be the nurse that is committed to her job, for the love, care and compassion of it.

I hope that's given you some food for thought to take with you to an interview in case they ask the question. Now back to interviews! Here are some tips and advice:

Tip: Write out a list of potential questions and give them to a friend or family member to ask you. Try to do a few practice runs to the place where your interview is before the day. This will avoid any lateness and put your mind at ease.

Another tip someone else gave me was, answer your interview questions in the mirror to yourself, which really helps too. ☺

What sort of questions will they ask you? From my own experience and from other student experiences that I have heard, you may be given a mixture of questions, scenarios and even a group discussion or presentation to do on the day. Some universities have an English and Maths exam before your interview but not all of them as some universities have started to remove these now from the interview process (unless you are an international student and then you may have this exam to assess you).

- Maths and English exams to start with are usually set at level 2. These aren't too bad so please don't worry too much. There are some great practice tests online for free, please have a search for them. I used GSCE bitesize online which helped me a lot!
- You might get a group discussion. This is where you will sit in a group with a few other students and be given a topic to talk about. This is to see your communication skills and how you communicate with other people in a group. It's important to listen and acknowledge others as well as having your own voice.
- Some universities may give you a topic to talk about on the day, so do some research around this topic and think outside the box! Always give the pros and cons of something to show you can look at something from different perspectives as this is something you will do in your assignments with 'critical analysis'.
- Know your 6 C's of nursing – Care, Compassion, Courage, Commitment, Communication and Competence. They may ask you to explain a couple of them and give examples of them and how you put them into practice.
- You may be asked what recent news articles you have read or heard about related to nursing and what you think about them.
- RELAX! I know it's hard, but just breathe, smile and do this. Someone told me, 'You are here out of the thousands of applications they had. They have picked you for an interview, they have seen something in you! Be proud of that, and don't forget, you're interviewing them too. Why should you choose them over your other applications?' This really helped me to relax on the day.
- Also, go to Facebook groups and twitter and ask if anyone has had an interview at the university you have yours at. They can give you more specific advice for each university. See Box 2.2 for questions you might be asked in your interview.

This is your chance to shine and show your passion for nursing. Don't be modest and make sure you sell yourself! Remember, if you don't sell yourself enough, that could be the extra point you needed to get a place over someone else – so go sell yourself and sell yourself well.

BOX 2.2 ■ Questions You Could Be Asked in an Interview

You might be asked:

1. Why you want to do nursing.
2. What qualities you can bring to nursing.
3. Your 5-year plans/goals.
4. What does dignity/diversity/advocate/empathy mean to you?
5. What's the difference between a healthcare assistant/student nurse and a qualified nurse?
6. Name two of the 6 C's and give examples of how you would do these in practice.
7. Nursing is tough, the workload can be high: How will you manage your workload?
8. Scenario – You have an angry family member on the ward, how would you handle that situation?
9. Scenario – A patient is refusing to wash every single day. What do you do?
10. Scenario – A patient does not want treatment, but the family are getting angry and adamant to listen to them that the patient should have the treatment. What would you do?
11. You make a drug error. How would you handle this?

Think of your communication skills, team working skills, autonomy, caring, delegation, empathy, dignity when answering questions too.

You will more than likely get some scenarios to answer. Some things around this to consider on these types of questions are confidentiality, body language, communication, maintaining patient dignity, empathy, safety of yourself/ patients, best interest of the patient and always seek help if you need it – *Good luck!!*

Skills for Nursing

I wanted to add a little bit about qualities and skills you need for nursing which might help with your interviews but also what's expected of you. In the demand of this role, you will need several skills. You will need to be flexible, organised and be able to prioritise your workload. You will also need great observation skills and be able to assess and respond to deteriorating patients (NHS, n.d.). In addition, the NHS also suggests you need wider skills of being caring, good communicator, be able to manage, use your judgement and to teach and advise others. The role of the nurse has greatly developed, and people are living longer with a variety of complex comorbidities. As a nurse, you need the skills to be able to meet the changes and the increase in complexity of the patient (King College, 2019).

I have an old nursing book called *British Red Cross Society nursing manual no. 2* dated 1939 (Parson, 1939). It was a gift from an old friend who had stumbled across it and thought I would love it and they were right! I love looking at the history of nursing and how it started. It's got some funny pages about the nurse duties needed to be a nurse which I wanted to add here, to show the evolution and demands of the nurse. Nurse duties in 1939 included: Be kind and sympathetic to the patient, to retore health of the patient but also to show firmness when needed. The nurse should act with understanding and in a way that does not distress a patient. They should also never discuss patient confidentiality with another person. Nurses must show loyalty to their doctor and keep accurate records. Nurses were not allowed to undermine any doctor in the presence of another person. Nurses should also keep quiet for the patient, and visitors are not allowed whilst a patient rests or has treatments. And finally, the nurse must maintain her well-being: mentally and physically. In addition, the book provides duties such as cleaning the room, floors, making beds and how to do this, how to cook and prepare food for a patient, bath and dress wounds for patients (Parson, 1939). The foundation of nursing that is stated, we still use today. However, there is more to the role now than these skills. The assessments of our patients are far more complex now with different medical conditions and the doctors listen to their nurse and ask for their advice on the patient. Not only that, but today, nurses can further their knowledge and become nurse prescribers or advance nurse practitioners or even Doctor of Nursing with a PhD.

My own personal opinion of what skills do you need – yes, all of the above. But for me the two that stand out are communication and care within the 6 C's. Because when these lack, the care provided to your patient goes wrong. Furthermore, you do need to be very emotionally resilient because you need to recognise your own emotions to prevent burn out as a nurse which we will discuss in the mental health section. In addition, it depends on what area of nursing you go into as to what skills you need. Each area has its own set of skills that you will need to learn. But as long as you have that foundation set, the rest you can train, gain more knowledge with time and practice.

SOME OF MY TOP ESSENTIALS TO HELP YOU WHEN YOU START UNIVERSITY (UNI)

This is one of the most common questions I get asked from students: '*What should I buy to help me get started at university?*' As a student nurse, the very first thing you are going to need is stationery, depending on what sort of person you are. This is the sort of person I am: I have stationery upon stationery and I love it! I just love stationery, I love writing in different colours, I love doing diagrams, I love doing pictures and I love to do doodles. It all helps with my revision and my memory as well, so I love to use like a huge variety of different stationery, different techniques to help me revise. However, if you don't like all the colours and things then you can literally just buy a pen and paper, that's fine too. If your way of learning is just basic pen-to-paper notes, that's ok – do what will help YOU.

I also bought a large pad that had different dividers inside it, so I could put different modules in each section. It's great to keep all of your notes in one place and it was really cheap from a cheap shop, so have a look around and don't over-spend – it's not needed. You are on a student budget, so you need to save money. Some people also like to use a Dictaphone, or you can get a voice recording app on your phone and it's completely free, so that you can record your lessons to listen back to it later and do your notes. Ask permissions first.

The next tip is to get yourself a diary. It's fine if you want to use your phone calendar to put things into your phone calendar as well so that you have always got it all on you. I really like to keep a diary with all of my plans in so I can write my work commitments, I can write my bank shifts, I can work out my placement hours and every lecture, any extracurricular activities and just every-thing goes into my diary. This helps to know where I'm at and what I'm doing. It's the best way to stay organised and that is one of the top tips for started nursing is to stay organised. Literally, prioritise everything. Organise your life and just be on the ball and you're going to be amazing! Another really common question I get asked a lot is, '*What books do I need for university?*' I'm just going to put out a small disclaimer here as always: it very much depends on what university you are going to as they might expect different things from you. However, just from my own experiences and a couple of other universities they don't necessarily expect you to buy books, but they do give you reading lists and suggestions of books that you can buy to help you with revision, assignments, things like that but I personally am not a book person. I haven't picked up one single physiology book throughout my time at university. Because for me, with anatomy and physiology I preferred to go through all my lecture plans and then I revised from the Khan Academy on YouTube, which is a fantastic resource as it makes it really simple and easy to understand. But again, go with caution with that as they do sometimes go a little bit too in-depth, and you don't need that extra in-depth stuff. They might also use different words as a lot of it is American, so, just be careful with that too. But I love the Khan Academy and honestly, they are the best YouTube channel that I have found to learn anatomy and physiology from. They have also got a website that you can use, and they have online quizzes and things like that. But back to the books. If you want a book, I recommend firstly checking your university and local library for them. Rent them for free. You can also look on social media pages as nurses give away their old books for free too! I did have a couple of very good books which did help me. One was a medications book (new guide to medicines and drugs) which showed the physiology of how the medications worked in the body. And then the British National Formulary (BNF) which is our medica-tions 'BIBLE'. EVERY single healthcare professional uses this. I personally wanted my own so I went to my local pharmacy and asked for any old BNF they had that I could have. Which they gave me for free. My advice here is, go to your local pharmacy, say you're a student nurse and if they have any old copies of BNFs you can have for your studies, and they should give you one if they have one. There is also the BNF app for your phone which is free too, but I personally love having the BNF in physical form to flick through. However, err on the side of caution about getting your phone out if you have the app when you're out on placement. There are some strict rules about using your mobile phone and if you're really desperate to look something up make sure it's okay with your mentor and you say, 'Listen, this is what I'm doing I'm just looking this up on the BNF app, is that okay?' and they shouldn't have a problem with that but just be cautious with that. My next book is not a necessity but I absolutely adore this book. It is called the 'student nurses guide to successful reflection.' However, I'm a little bit biased because this is actually one of the lectures at Birmingham City University book, but she's fantastic and the way this book is set out is just incredible. If you struggle with reflection like I did at the start of university then this book is going to help you. There are different little tasks inside for you to do and you just go and work along the tasks. It is really helpful and it's got amazing quotes and things inside the book. It's really cute. It's just really simple and easy to understand. It is a broken-down book on reflection and how to do a real reflection. That's really helped me because as nurses we have to reflect – it's not even an option, it's mandatory and it's an NMC requirement as part of the revalidation process that you have to write reflections. So, you're going to need some sort of reflection tool, but it is 100% worth it. Have a look at it as it's fantastic. But if you don't want to spend money because we don't get paid for the nursing degree, have a look on search engines for different reflection tools as there's loads of free online step-by-step guides on how to reflect. There are different tools that you can use to help you reflect and you don't really need to buy a book.

What bag to get for university? Yet another common question, so here we are. For me, I am obsessed with backpacks. I love backpacks and they're great for placement and they are great for university. I have about seven backpacks (four for university) and I rotate them all. So, my main backpack I use just for placements is absolutely massive! And you need a bigger bag for placement because you're going to need to put your uniform in there (because you can't wear your uniform travelling to and from placement and you have to get changed at placement) and I need to also put all of the food in there for the day too. Mine also had a little pouch to put things such as your laptop or your placement documents in to keep them safe. It was one of my favourites and a bargain! I got this from Costco and it was around 10 pounds. But my other backpacks are just slightly smaller and I use them for university just to put my pens and paper, lunch, things like that in. Get whichever bag you want but just make sure it's comfortable and make sure it fits all your things in. Also, make sure it's practical, you don't need an expensive bag, as long as it does the job. It's not a fashion show.

My next essential item for student nursing (and it REALLY IS essential you have this) is to get yourself a fob watch. You will need this, and it is 100% mandatory because you need this when you go out to placement and you're doing observation checks and you need to count respiratory rates or for counting the pulse rate. Preferably, you should get the ones in a rubber case because they're washable and these you can get online cheap. So have a look around as you can get some for a few pounds.

My next essential is to get yourself a pocket note pad because as you go along on your placements, your mentor is going to be telling you things or other nurses or the doctors, consultants, health care assistants etc., are going to be giving you all of this information and it's really good to just jot things down. I also put my medications in there because throughout university you'll be given a set number of medications to learn, so I literally just write all of my medications in there as well. I tend to keep the front for medications and then the back for any information advice. And it's good to look back on and just read up on your notes, or if you forget something you can refer back to your note pad instead of keep asking your mentor the same things.

On the subject of placements you need comfy shoes! Another MUST HAVE item. And you need the ugliest and the most horrible looking ones (because they are usually the comfiest haha!) Shoes for placement must be wipeable and they have to cover your whole foot, so they can't be like dolly shoes with gaps. They're going to need to be wipeable because you're going to get body fluids on them; you're going to get blood, you're going to get urine and you're going to get vomit on there. So, you're going to want to be able to wipe them. Many students get their shoes from Clarks – I had the 'unloop' ones and they were just the comfiest things I've ever worn. However, I did also get given a free pair of shoes from a company called Toffeln online. They are specialists in making nursing shoes and I still wear them today! They were created by a university and researchers and come with different insoles depending on your foot shape. Just amazing! They can be pricey, but they were so worth it, and I have had mine for over 2 years, and they still look brand new. I just can't believe I didn't get them sooner. I got these as a newly qualified nurse. If you go to somewhere like Clarks, they are also a bit pricey if you go into the regular shop, I think they're about 60 pounds. So, please, any advice that you take from this go to the factory outlet or online sales because these are like half the price in the outlet. I got mine for 35 pounds I think at the factory outlet. Please, save your money but also some students have commented saying that they don't like wearing these shoes and that they found them uncomfortable. They just can't adjust to them, and they opted for Sketchers instead but it's up to you, just go out there and try on shoes. Do not look for a fashionable look, like I said, it's not a fashion show and they will get ruined. Go for the ugliest, safest, cleanest and comfiest shoes that you can find, because you're on your feet for twelve and a half hours and you are going to need comfy shoes.

Another thing that I have bought is a manual blood pressure set and I got this really cheap online – it was 5 pounds. Because as a nurse you're going to have to do manual blood pressure. On the wards you've got electric blood pressure machines but there will be times that you might have to use a manual blood pressure. I know in our very first OSCE exam we are tested on manual blood pressure, so it's good to have that at home to just practice on people, on your friends, your family, your animals if you want, but it just really helps build your confidence with manual blood pressure. I know some people do struggle when they're doing it, so it's good to have this but again you don't 100% need that, that's just something I wanted to practice at home. Mainly because I loved it and I love doing manual blood pressure. But there will be things at your university to help you practice that so don't go spending the money that you don't have and it's not a necessity, it's just something that I prefer to have.

My final essential, last but not least, mainly for when you're out on placement is a good hand cream. When you are washing your hands every single day, all day, you are going to get extremely sore, cracked and dry skin, so just have a really good hand cream in your bag. A small one that can go in your pocket is always good as well, because your hands do get dry, and they do get sore. It is a really big thing because you must look after yourself and you have to look after your hands. There are so many different hand creams to choose from, so go with whatever suits your skin and that is going to protect them all day long. Whichever hand cream you choose, just make sure it's a good one for your hands. So that's my top essentials you're going to need as a nursing student, I hope it helps.

FUN FACT

Did you know that there are 301,491 nurses working within the NHS alone, whilst there are only around 123,813 doctors (DOH, 2021).

References

Collins Dictionary. (2020). *Definition of plagiarism.* Retrieved from https://www.collins-dictionary.com/dictionary/english/plagiarism. Accessed 14 September 2020.

DOH. (2021). *Record number of NHS doctors and nurses in England.* Retrieved from https://www.gov.uk/government/news/record-number-of-nhs-doctors-and-nurses-in-england. Accessed 16 May 2022.

Kings College. (2019). *Skills that meet the needs of all who access healthcare: Why nursing higher education is essential.* Retrieved from https://www.kcl.ac.uk/news/why-nursing-higher-education-is-essential. Accessed 16 May 2022.

NHS. (n.d.). *Personal characteristics and skills required (adult nursing).* Retrieved from https://www.healthcareers.nhs.uk/explore-roles/nursing/roles-nursing/adult-nurse/personal-characteristics-and-skills-required-adult-nursing. Accessed 16 May 2022.

NHS England. (2015). *Introducing the 6C's.* London: NHS. Retrieved from https://www.england.nhs.uk/6cs/wp-content/uploads/sites/25/2015/03/introducing-the-6cs.pdf . Accessed 21 September 2021.

Oxford Dictionary. (n.d.). *Care*. Retrieved from https://www.oxfordlearnersdictionaries. com/definition/american_english/care_1. Accessed 27 May 2022.

Parson, H. C. (1939). *British Red Cross Society nursing manual no.2* (5th ed., pp. 4–7). London: HK Lewis & Co. Ltd.

UCAS. (2020a). *Advisor guide 2020*. Retrieved from https://www.ucas.com/file/225446/ download?token=V_k10YE8. Accessed 14 September 2020.

UCAS. (2020b). *How to write a UCAS undergraduate personal statement*. Retrieved from https://www.ucas.com/undergraduate/applying-university/how-write-ucas-under-graduate-personal-statement. Accessed 14 September 2020.

CHAPTER 3

What to Do in Your First Few Weeks of University

With a Case Study From Dawn Jones (a Student and a Mother)

Congratulations, You Are In!

You have bagged that university place, and it's leading up to your first days/ weeks. This feeling was full of excitement for me! I couldn't wait to get started but I was going alone, I didn't have any friends and this was a huge anxiety of mine at the start. People see my YouTube videos, social media and think of me as this big extrovert – but I'm the complete opposite. I like my home comforts, I don't like big crowds of people and even worse, people I don't know and having to make small talk: it all makes me extremely anxious (although I am way better at it now). This is weird because as a nurse, I am completely different, and I always love talking with patients and making time for them. It never seems as scary for some reason. What made my experience worse was, there was an administration error on my application, and no one had told me the start date or time or anything. When I called to get this information, they informed me that the course had started the previous week! I had missed out on inductions, meeting new people, and making connections.

On my first day, I was full of nerves, I remember standing outside the door to the room I needed to be in and kept thinking, everyone knows each other already, how do I make friends now?! And to be quite honest, I sat alone for the first couple of months! Don't get me wrong, I tried to speak to people, I just failed. I remember deciding to sit next to someone, and I tried to speak to them, but they completely blanked me! Another person I sat next to, we got along so well, and chatted etc., and then at the end of the lecture they just got up and left – didn't even say goodbye. Left me heartbroken. So, I sat alone until one day whilst I was standing in the coffee shop line, someone came up to me and said, 'Do you want to come and sit with us?' And I did, and I never left them haha. They became my circle of friends for the next (almost) 3 years of university and we all keep in contact now that we have all qualified. So, my first tip is, make friends, speak to people, sit next to people and do all you can to make friends. Push yourself out of that comfort zone because that is how you'll grow. If you

---

BOX 3.1 ■ Checklist for Your First Few Weeks at University

- Have you completed, signed and submitted all your finance applications?
- Have you had your occupational health appointment at university?
- Do you have your start date? If not, call the university school office in case there has been a glitch in the system.
- Do you have everything you need for university? Pens, paper, fob watch, shoes etc.?
- Do you have your accommodation arranged if you're moving out?
- If you are an international student or new to the area, have you registered with a doctor/general practitioner (GP)? The university can help with this.
- Get your head around the room numbers and locations. Do a walk around the university to get yourself orientated to the layout of rooms.
- Take time to find your feet around the university.
- Download and print your yearly planner.
- Download and print your exam/assignment timetable and prioritise what comes first.
- Check out what events are going on at your university and take part (optional) – this will help you get to know other people.
- Make the most of extracurricular activities outside your nursing studies – this will take your mind off deadlines and keep you motivated (optional).
- Don't forget to take some time out for YOU. This course can be intense, and you will need the support of your family and friends as well as alone time to rest and recharge.
- Email and meet your personal tutor. They are your first point of call if you need anything, along with the module leaders, and they do your reference at the end of your degree for your first nursing job.
- Have a look around your library and ask for an induction on how to get books and use their website etc.
- The library also can help you look for articles and journals for your assignments.
- If you don't know something, ask and don't be scared to put your hand up! More than likely, everyone else is thinking the same thing.
- If you're struggling, please talk to someone – friends, personal tutor, lecturer. Your university might have a counselling service you can access too. Just make sure you get the help you need. Never suffer in silence.

---

have friends, make new friends, watch out for the ones who are sitting alone – say hello and smile. This is the next 3 years of your life; those friends are going to be the support group you need to keep you motivated and on the ball.

So, what important things should you be doing in your first few weeks at university (other than making friends) (Box 3.1)?

A Piece From Dawn Jones – Second-Year Student Nurse (At the Time of Writing This)

First of all, congratulations on becoming a student nurse, and having children while doing your studies. It is such a great achievement.

As a student nurse and mum to three daughters (16 years old, 9 years old and 5 years old), it can be a challenge and you may be feeling overwhelmed, with having to balance family life, university and having to attend placements.

When starting university, it can seem very daunting learning everything and trying to figure out what you need get into place. Even more worries that you have children to organise as well. If your children attend school, you can ask them if they have breakfast or after-school clubs that may help. (Your funding unit at the university may help with the costs; seek this information as soon as possible.) Another person who can help with information or advice is your Advisor of Studies/Academic Advisor. They can keep you on the right path with your studies, and they are more than happy to help.

I know from my experience, I have sought guidance from my lecturers and my Advisor of Studies to help and give me advice on things myself and my family have gone through. They have always given me time to express myself and discussed private matters when I needed to. So please use your university resources when you need that support. They are there to be used, they can help.

If you have a learning disability, make sure you contact your disability services to get things into place before starting your course. Always plan to get the most out of your time at university. This service is one to use if you need that little extra support and will help you have a great experience. I am dyslexic and have Meares Irlen's (visual eye stress). My disability services have put things into place for me when I require them (e.g. 15 minutes added to exams, one-to-one study support).

As I have mentioned before, making the most of what your university can help you with makes your experience flow smoother and with the children, a natural routine will follow. It will be hard to begin with, but trust me it does get easier. Planning, routines, sharing hints and tips with other students will all help you find what works best for you and your family.

Another thing to mention, if you can, getting into the National Health Service (NHS) bank healthcare support worker is another good way to help start making new friends and getting to know your way around your local hospital. I really do enjoy working at the bank. It keeps me involved with learning so many new things, as does being on a university placement. Just remember if you do, work within your different roles/limitations. But it is a great experience for yourself, not just to be mum, it's a break away from home life and be our own person for a few hours.

A little about myself. Currently, I am a 2nd year nursing student (in Scotland). I live with my husband and my three daughters. We are also a military family, and this can be difficult to juggle. My eldest struggles with mental health, my middle daughter is awaiting a diagnosis of attention deficit hyperactivity disorder (ADHD) and my youngest is autistic. Balancing these concerns and university life does have its challenges for me, but it is rewarding to be able to have this opportunity to become the nurse I've always wanted. I couldn't do this without the support of my husband, kids, dad and aunt, and my amazing friends along the way.

Be proud of what you're going to achieve, or what you already are achieving, making new friends, your kids making new friends along with you. Studying and being on placement is such a rewarding experience, the patients you get to help and meet are amazing.

Something to know and remind ourselves: there will be tears and stresses, days when you want to give up, but please remember you're doing this course to become a nurse, one your children will be proud of. Not only are we advocates for our patients, but we are also providing a future for our children.

Below are just some things I feel that might help other student nurses studying and having a family:

- It is important to know there is help for you at university for parents. Get to know what's available to you within the resources, for example, some universities have nurseries on campus or can help find a nursery within your area.
- Seek out new friends from university that have children as well. It's good to have someone who knows what it's like going through the same experiences. You can confide in each other and even have play dates for your children.
- When trying to study, if you have your children at home, give them some tasks that they can do while you're busy. This could be anything from drawing some art or, depending on their age, homework to complete.
- Having a good routine for yourself and your children is always a great idea. The children will find this useful as well as yourself.
- If possible, ask for help from family and friends. Having good support around you is important, as they can help with the children and give you a little break to get some studying done. (I know not many people have this kind of support, but any help is great).
- I am a big believer in, when my girls head to bed, allowing myself at least 1 hour of study (better than none, anything helps).
- For my girls, I have given them each their own spaces at home so that they can have their alone time (we all need our own space and to minimise any sibling arguing).
- What I find works for me is making a list for everything (very simple I know but trust me it does wonders). This helps me a lot as I can keep track of what I need to do each day and which daughter I need to take to an appointment etc. (if there is any).
- Learn from me, always start your essays/assignments as soon as you can. I have had times I've left things to last minute and it is not worth the stress. Plan, plan and plan!!
- A good idea is to prep the children's clothes/school bags for the next day. This saves time in the morning, and you can get out the door quicker. This is a massive time saver for my family.

- Get outside and have a break if you're online learning with university, especially if you have young children at home. It's great for your mental health and helps the children to use up their energy.

I started university the year of the nurse – 2020 – as COVID was happening. So, the majority of my learning has been online, and now, again, with visits to the university. So being out on placement has been an amazing experience. Meeting other students as well as assessors and supervisors.

Thank you

Student Nurse Dawn

FUN FACT

Ninety-five per cent of the population said nursing was the most trusted profession compared with others such as teachers or salespeople (ID Medical, 2022).

References

ID Medical. (2022). *10 amazing facts about nursing*. Retrieved from https://www.id-medical.com/10-amazing-facts-about-nursing/. Accessed 19 May 2022.

CHAPTER 4

Assignment Help

One thing I worried about before starting university was assignments and how to even write them! I wasn't academic at all, and this was causing me a lot of anxiety starting off. Firstly, don't panic! It's not as bad as it all seems honestly. I didn't have a clue to start with, my assignment was as basic as it could get, and I still passed. I didn't use fancy wording; I didn't go into huge amounts of detail, and I still got 55%. To be honest, even though this was a pass it was a low grade, and I was gutted. I knew I wouldn't do well but when it hits you like that, it makes you realise just how much you want to improve. Not only that, but going into the second and third years, the marking criteria goes up, which means I needed to level up too. I read all of the feedback, visited my personal development department and received all the help I could get for writing my second assignment. Never be ashamed to ask for help, trust me, it all helps.

I then went on to get 75% for my second and third assignments!! I was so happy! All I did was a few small changes that I was advised and managed to get such a great grade. I want to share with you what I did to help me achieve higher. I am going to just say this again, it all depends on where you are in the world and what university you are studying at. ***Please check your own university guidelines, assignment brief and marking criteria and go against that over anyone else's advice on this.*** These will also give you guidance and what to aim for to get higher grades if that's what you want. However, this book won't get you the grades, your hard work, determination, blood sweat, and tears will get you that grade: If you write the assignment well, you'll get the results. If it's not a well-written assignment and you don't cover what they expect you to, you will fail. So please, I can't stress this enough – read the assignment brief, and make sure you can tick off everything it is asking of you on the assignment brief before anything else. This is the main tip I always followed to pass, so I hope it helps you. And if you don't understand your assignment brief, contact your tutor or the module lead/lecturer and get them to explain it to you. You can also use the library staff as well to help with this. But like I said, every university is different, I am very fortunate that at my university, they had a few things in place like a personal development department that helped with these things.

Firstly, you want a structure, like with all assignments you need: an introduction, a main body and then a conclusion.

Nottingham University (n.d.) discuss the four types of writers by Créme and Lea, which are:

1. **The Diver** – This is me… I dive right into the assignment with no plan. Whenever I try and plan, it never works. I'm far better and just putting pen to paper (or finger to laptop)

2. **The Patchwork Writer** – Someone that starts with headings/subheadings and builds from there but will also move from one section to another. I have also done this; I like to create subheadings from an assignment brief to make sure I do everything that is required to pass.

3. **The Architect** – Is the master planner! They have a clear plan of what they want to do before even starting. They will make notes and guides to help them.

4. **The Grand Plan Writer** – This is someone who reads A LOT before starting their writing. They read and read and then when they have enough information to mind, they write, and it will flow from there (Nottingham University, n.d.)

I mention these things as it's really important to work out what style you have. Next, where do you work best? What type of environment helps get that brain flowing? For me, it was my dining room. I lived in a shared house at the time, and when I sat in my own room, I found I got so distracted by TV and social media. But the minute I moved to the dining room I could focus well. It really is amazing what an environment does for you. Move around your house and university to find your comfort zone for working. This will help you with future assignments and enable you to work to the best of your ability. However, if you have a lot of distractions, you won't be able to work. This can also be hard for students who have young children. So, for you, it's about finding the best time, when the children are not around, to do the work.

I also discovered something amazing, and this was Google Books. If you go onto google.com and search for the book you want to. Let's just say, for example, you want to find more about resilience, it'll come up with a whole load of books on resilience and not only that if you click into these books, but you can also actually read a lot more of the book than normal. If you go into Amazon and things, they give you little snippets of the book may be one page or two pages just so you can kind of take a sneak peek inside but some of these give you the whole book to read. So, then you don't even really have to take a step inside a library to take out the book. You can read through the book, it's there in the comfort of your own home. You can take out any key parts that you want to take from the book and put them into your assignments and then you can reference it the same as you would reference a book. Because you've got all the information there is as if you've got the book in your hands, it's just an online version. But I must say in assignment writing it is far better to look up journal articles and use a lot more evidence-based practice and journal articles over books with your reference in because they're seen as the best evidence possible. So, if you want high marks go for more journal articles over books with your references.

The University of Nottingham (2014) has a great guide on writing assignments, one part, they share is how to process words written on an assignment brief. This is THE hardest part of assignment writing I found. It all looked like random words thrown together that just didn't make any sense to me. I often had to Google words to figure out what was expected of me to be able to start writing. I'm not sure why universities do this? Why can't they just put things into simple English to understand? If this is you, then, the table below is for you, I hope this helps break it down a little bit. These are some of the common words you may see and what they mean/how the university expects you to write your assignment (Table 4.1).

Some of my other tips I can give for writing assignments are:

- Use linking words in your assignment to make it flow nicely. This was one of the biggest tips I received, and it really helped me. There is a fantastic website called Manchester Phrase bank, look at that (other sites are available). However, here are a few to get you started (Table 4.2)
- Use evidence-based practice, research papers and more journal articles rather than books. This was the second biggest tip I was given. **Rationale behind this**: As nurses, we must work on evidence-based practice when out in the real world with real patients. It shows that we have done our research and put the evidence into our own practice. This ensures patient safety, and we can provide the patient with the best care possible using the most up-to-date evidence available (Lehane et al., 2019).
- Always follow your assignment brief and marking criteria and avoid listening to other people's comments on what to include in your assignment. You don't know who will be marking your assignment and all they have in front of them will be your assignment brief and the marking criteria.
- Write about what you love! If you have a choice of subjects to choose from, write the one that appeals to you the most. If you write about what you love, this assignment will become easy and enjoyable to write. Don't make it harder for yourself. I remember one of my friends decided to write about something new and random just to gain more knowledge – which is a great idea. However, he made it so much harder for himself as a result.
- I personally put in a reference every 50 to 55 words. But references should always come after any statement you make and use references from different, reliable but good quality sources such as journals, and government documents and do **NOT** reference google. We are nurses and need to follow reliable and legit sources for our information and not just some random website. This will also show you have a wider reading of the topic and will bag yourself some extra marks.
- Break your assignment down into small manageable pieces. This will make this so much easier to write. I use subheadings to help me separate what I'm writing and then remove them and add linking words to help it flow

TABLE 4.1 ■ Common Assignment Abbreviations

Account for	Give reasons for something or explain why something is happening
Analyse	Examine something critically, identify the main points of something and any significant events of something – do so in great detail
Assess	To identify and weigh up the value of something
Comment on	Identify the main problem, show the evidence to support your points made – NOT personal opinions.
Compare	Showing similarities/strengths of two or more things. Also showing the important areas too of these.
Contrast	Showing the opposites/weaknesses of two or more things. But also showing the relevance and importance of them.
Compare and contrast	Showing both of the above
Criticise	Creating a judgement based on evidence about something. Use examples and evidence-based practice to back up this.
Critically evaluate	Weighing up the weaknesses and strengths for something. Providing an argument for and against and show evidence of why you have written this.
Define	Show the exact meaning of something. There can be more than one and you can write about what you agree/disagree with too.
Describe	Show the main features of something and write a detailed account of something.
Discuss	Explain and talk about/arguments for and against something. Show evidence of this.
Distinguish/ differentiate	Finding differences between something
Evaluate	Assessing something's worth, effectiveness and supported by evidence. Weighing up for and against again.
Examine	Looking at something in more detail
Explain	You will explain why something happens or the way it happens
How far	Looking at evidence or arguments and weighing them up.
Illustrate	Using examples to explain something clearly and explicitly.
Interpret	Showing the meaning of something in more detail
Justify	Show why you have made a decision about something based on evidence you have gathered
Narrate	This focuses on the series of events and what has happened
Outline	Giving the main points of the topic
Relate	Similarities/connections between two or more things
State	Write the main features of something: keeping it clear and brief
Summarise	Writing the main points of something: again, clear and brief
To what extent	Weighing up how convincing something is. Is it true? How far?

TABLE 4.2 ■ Linking Words

Adding to a Sentence/ Point	Comparing/ Giving an Example	Contrasting Words	Conse- quence	Concluding
Furthermore	In comparison	However	Therefore	Overall
Moreover	For example	In contrast	Thus	To summarise
In addition	Firstly, sec- ondly, lastly	On the other hand	As a consequence	To conclude
Similarly	Clearly	Unlike	As a result	In conclusion
Not only did... but also...	In the same way For instance	Nonetheless Nevertheless	For that reason Hence	Finally In brief
What is more	To illustrate To demonstrate	Although	Consequently Despite this Accordingly	

before submitting. Chip away at it slowly and it will all come together nicely in no time.

- Less is more! This sounds bizarre but let me explain. If you have numerous things to discuss in your assignment, narrow it down to one or two or even three and then go in-depth with them. For example, if you're writing about consent, there are so many types of consent. Just pick one or two types and go in-depth with them. Look at what you *need* to write and don't over-complicate it.
- Reference as you go. I personally don't leave referencing to the last minute. I write my piece and then go and find the reference to back up what I am saying. I will input the citation into the main body and then the reference list there and then. This saves so much time at the end of the assignment. It is also frustrating if you can't find any evidence to back up what you are saying, so this saves time later.
- Be critical in your assignment – That's where the good marks are at. This is level 5 and 6 markings; I have a page dedicated to critically analysing (see this section for more)

I hope this has given you enough to start thinking about how to write your assignment and hopefully pass! Good luck to you all.

Dissertation Help

I couldn't write an assignment help chapter without including the dreaded dissertation! Disclaimer, some universities do not have a dissertation, and these are called other things in different areas. Please check with your university on what they do and how they do it before taking any advice onboard.

Hopefully I'm going to be able to help and put your mind at rest on dissertations and hopefully give you some advice and tips to help you get through it. Firstly, I just wanted to say that dissertation was something that I, personally, really panicked about. It was something I've always panicked about so much so that it almost made me not come to do my nursing degree. Because I was so paranoid, worried, and anxious about the dissertation and how I'm going to manage to write so well, and I wasn't academic at all. All these fears have been going around my head for a long time before I even started nursing. Until I made the leap but worried throughout the first and second years about this. In my second year, I actually started to research my topic ready for my dissertation because I was so worried about it, and I wanted to be prepared as much as I could be. So, I can fully understand your anxieties and worries right now I promise you, but you know what? I got through it, and I've done it and actually… it was alright, I'm alive and well I was smiling at the end of it because I knew it was done. However, the process of doing it is hard, it is very long-winded, and you will tear your hair out and it might even drain your soul a little bit… (not to scare you). But overall, it's okay and it's not too bad at all really when I think back to it now. For me personally, it was because I'm so organised and I like to get an assignment done and dusted. But this is something that you physically can't do with a dissertation. I can't but hats off to you if you can do that. I physically can't sit down and write a whole dissertation in a night or even a week, this has taken me a whole year to do.

So, my dissertation was a dissertation/not called dissertation… They changed the wording, and it was called: Academic and Practice Enquiry (AcPE) instead which was a 4000-word literature review. We had to come up with our own research question using a Population/Problem/Patient; Intervention/Issue; Comparison; Outcome (PICO) or a Population/Problem/Patient, Exposure, Outcome (PEO). Then once we found our literature, we had to use a CASP tool (Critical Appraisal Skills Programme), which is used to critically appraise and show the strengths and weaknesses of every single article (CASP, 2022). I had to do ten of those, one for each article, and then once I found all the strengths and weaknesses, I put all of that into a data extraction table. Then once I had done this data extraction table, I had to create a theme table. Then once I had done the theme table, I found reoccurring themes within all of the articles which then correspond to the answer to the question. Then I go into my results section and conclusion and things like that so that's overall, what we did. That's a really Whistlestop tour of what we had to do for our AcPE.

What I discovered was that 4000 words were just not enough, so I used tables, I had to use appendices and things like that to sort of help me out a little bit. It was quite tough to narrow it all down because everything I was writing, needed to be in there. That was by far, my toughest challenge with that. I just wanted to give an overview of what we had to do, however, again, this might be different to your university. And your university will give you all of the information and how to complete your dissertation (or another name). So don't panic about this right now, please.

Here are my main top tips for you to start your dissertation and I'm going to make it broad, top tips so that whatever you're doing your dissertation on, however you do your dissertation, it's just going to be tips that are going to help you hopefully. My first tip is always my tip for everything, to be organised! Look at this as early as possible and it is never too soon to start looking at your dissertation. As I said, I started mine in my second year where I started researching around the topic and thinking about possible questions for my topic and then I looked at research papers on my topic. It took me months and months and months to find my 10 papers for this. It took me a long time and the main bulk of your whole assignment is finding the research out there, so, get a head start and do that first before anything.

If you've got some time off over the summer, or Christmas, I know we all want to be out there having fun and making the most of our time off, but if you get a head start early, it's going to save you a lot, a lot of work in the third year I promise you. One question I get asked a lot is: 'when you're looking at your research articles, how do you know if it's good enough or not to use in your dissertation?' The best tip I can ever give, well, is not a tip, it's more advice. But this is what you're trying to assess within a literature review. I know our one was all about how to find a good quality piece of research that backs up what you're doing out there in nursing practice. This is your job and doing your literature review is working out if the article/research is good enough or not. This is where the use of your CASP tool comes in, so, if you have got an article that isn't very good quality and you've done your CASP and it shows a lot of weaknesses – that's great because that's critical, you are going to be able to critically analyse that amazingly in your result section. That's going to give you some massive brownie points so don't worry about it being a strong or weak article or research paper or whatever it is, if you can explain it and critique it, you're going to be well away. You're going to have those really strong articles that you found, and it is going to balance it and make it sound juicy hopefully.

If you're really struggling for articles, go to your local library or your personal development department and get them to help you search as well. Not only this but they can actually gain access to articles that you might not have access to. They can put in requests for articles for you to access if there's any restrictions in place. I've done this and it really helped me because it found my last tenth article. But please make use of all of the services at the university because that's what they're there and for they're free. It will just open a whole new world and hopefully, you'll be able to find your articles a lot faster.

My next tip is to make sure you want to write about something you're passionate about. You're going to be spending so long on this dissertation, like I said it's going to drain your soul. You want it to be something interesting, something juicy, something that you really want to look into and something that gets you excited. Think about what you've done so far in your nursing career or experienced out there as a healthcare assistant, anything like that and look at what you're interested in and what you want to know more about. Things that you can relate to practice and anything that's going to help in your job role. Have a look at where you want to work as well because you could do your dissertation on something related. Such as cardiac-related if you want to work in a cardiology world or if you want to do something about the chronic obstructive pulmonary disease (COPD) or lung cancer or respiratory problems because you want to work in a respiratory ward. If something really fascinates you, do your dissertation on that because that's going to give you massive brownie points when you go to your interview for your job. You can say 'I'm that interested in this area I've done my dissertation on it' – that's going to just blow their mind hopefully. Also, if you do something interesting, you will enjoy writing it and researching it and that's going to help you get through it.

My next tip is to break it down into small manageable sections. Because this is a lot of work and it's a massive word count. If you just break it down into manageable bite-size steps, it's going to be so much easier honestly. This is what I've done for all my assignments. I've just done all these sections bit by bit stage by stage and you'll come to the end, and you'll think looking at it 'I've actually done that and I've done that and I've actually not got as much as I thought that I had to do'. Because you'll be doing it as you go. Also, set yourself goals with it as well, use those specific, measurable, attainable, relevant and time-bound (SMART) goals that we have talked about in this book to help you get through this. I slowly chipped away at mine, and suddenly it was complete. You'll look back at it and go 'wow I'm finished' and it'll be the best feeling in the world I promise you.

What really helps is having a calendar as well. At our University, they made it easy for us and they gave us an actual schedule to complete each section within a certain time frame. So, between January to March was all about finding your research and getting your 10 articles together and then March till May with doing your CASP tools for your articles and then May to so-and-so was doing your introduction and all of that. They really broke it down amazingly for us, so if you can just get a calendar or create some form of timetable schedule for yourself that will help.

And a huge thank you to Birmingham City University for this! I'm not paid to say that I promise haha.

My next tip may be a little bit of a controversial one... but I'm going to say this anyway Google is your best friend right now! I know we are told never to google anything; however, if you're like me I don't understand research and I am NOT a fan of research. Because I didn't understand any of the terminology, I haven't got a clue still with some of it. I will sit and I will read articles and I'm reading it but it's not going in. I'm not used to this terminology, and I'm not used to this way of writing. So, Google did become my best friend and I googled every single word that I didn't understand, and it just really helped me. But alongside this tip of Google, use the phrase banks as well which I have already mentioned in the assignment section.

There are many books to help you write a dissertation as well if you want to use that. I personally, didn't read any books to help me and managed to pass without that.

My final last tip for you is to make the most of the supervision or your supervisors. You will be designated a supervisor for your dissertation, and you can go and ask for help or you can email them. Make the most of that time with them, have a one-to-one, write down a list of everything you want to know, everything you want to ask so that you don't forget when you're there. Because that's something I do all of the time; I'll go to a doctor or something (because I never go to the doctor) and I'll wait until I've got 101 things wrong with me (I'm a really bad patient) and I'll go in and I'll forget. As a result, I have learned to write down things whenever I go into meetings now or one-to-ones or tutorials. I have my list ready; I'm organised and prepared. And you can just go over everything, but please make use of them, they are there to guide you and to help you. They don't want to see you fail, so just make the most of that time with your supervisors.

I just wanted to say, lastly, dissertation was a massive scary thing that I had dreaded for years and years this goes back 10 years ago when I didn't want to do the degree because of the academic side. I wanted to do the diploma purely because I didn't want to face a dissertation, I worried about it all through my first year and then again in the second year. So, when it came to the point that I had finished my dissertation, it was like a huge weight had lifted off me. I realised it wasn't that bad. Ok, yeah, it was a little soul-draining because it takes a long time. But it wasn't as bad as I made out in my head. Don't get me wrong, you're going to struggle at times, you're going to tear your hair out and you're going to put posts on social media maybe, saying you're really sick of seeing this dissertation. But you WILL and CAN do this.

Trust me, if I can do a (kind of) dissertation, coming from a non-academic background or almost failing my General Certificate of Secondary Education (GCSEs), if I can get through this and write a dissertation (and I got a first for it!!) – so can you! So come on, put on your positivity pants, you can do this, go get started with what you're waiting for and good luck!

Data Base Searching

I know a lot of students struggle with database searching and I know I struggled a lot for the first two years. But I didn't know I was searching all wrong until I went to my university library and spoke to the librarian. I said 'do you know what? I'm searching these articles but it's not coming up with anything and I can't find anything. I can't find what I'm looking for, what am I doing wrong?' She literally showed me these couple of simple things and it just completely changed the way I searched forever! And just like that, I realised I had been doing it wrong all this time which affected my work. So, I hope this section will help other people out because I'm sure everybody is probably doing what I was doing and hopefully it's going to help you and this is going to make your assignment writing so much easier in the future, fingers crossed. I will talk you through it bit by bit on what to do using CINAHL (a database search engine).

The first thing that I just wanted to mention about database searching is to use a wide variety of different databases so go on to CINAHL, Cochrane library, MEDLINE and even Google Scholar to search for different journal articles or research papers. Have a look at those and start searching for the things you want to.

This is how I was originally searching for my articles; I opened CINAHL and went to the search bar and enter what I wanted to find, just a keyword (I was researching chlamydia as my main keyword). Then I went to the bar underneath this to add another keyword (Young people). I was searching chlamydia in the top bar and then underneath it I would type in the search bar *AND* 'young people' and then press search (Fig. 4.1)

Then I was just pressing search like that. But it was only coming up with a few results, I think it was about five results at the time. This is why I was stressing about it, because I knew chlamydia and sexual health in young people was a huge area with hundreds of research papers out there. But it was strange that nothing was coming up and I just couldn't believe that there was no research showing for it. That's when I decided to go into the library for help and then realised, I was searching all wrong. So, I am going to show you exactly what the librarian taught me, to hopefully help you out in future.

Firstly, you want to put your main search topic in the top bar and press search – but do NOT add anything else in the other boxes below (like I did…). So, for mine, I would just search chlamydia in the top box and nothing else, then press search. Then it comes up with A LOT of articles, I had thousands of results come up! So, now you want to narrow it down because you can't go through hundreds or thousands of papers, you just don't have time or the patience for that haha. But now you're going to do a new search on that same results page. So,

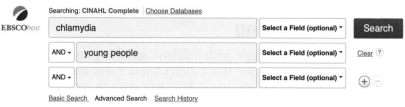

Fig. 4.1   Screen shot from CINAHL Complete (2022a).

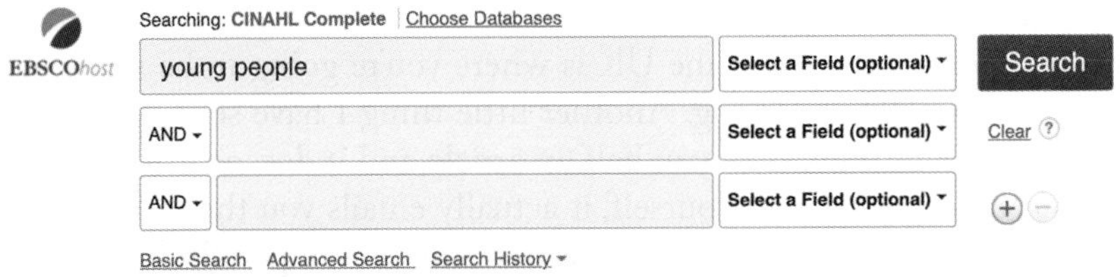

Fig. 4.2 CINAHL complete. Young people.

you will be inputting your next topic, so 'young people' was my second topic, so I entered this and pressed search again (Fig. 4.2). Images taken from CINAHL Complete (2022b).

Which came up with thousands of results for that one separately. So now we want to combine the two results together to narrow it down even more and be more specific for what you're looking for. So, you have to click on 'search history' which is just underneath your search bars (see Fig. 4.1 for this tab) and then tick on the left-hand side 'select all' and then the 'search with' tab (Fig. 4.3).

That will then combine the two together topics together and give you the accurate results for what you are looking for. Once I had combined these two, I then had 79 results to pick from which was better than just a few that I was getting before. Then you can just go through all your results and see if there are any articles there you can find. Also, you can add on searches so that instead of young people you might try, young adults or adolescents' teenagers instead, so it will do a wider search with those different keywords.

It's about finding different keywords and just searching each one till you find your best result. That's just the one main thing that I was going wrong with, I was literally searching completely wrong but just that small tweak, that small change, and it brings up better results, more results and it narrows it down. Also, on the side of the screen somewhere, you can pick geography, so you can pick the UK and narrow it down even more if you really want to. But just picking the UK, doesn't mean you're going to get just purely UK-based research. The researchers might be UK-based but the actual research they've taken might be in a different country, such as the USA, Japan, India, or somewhere like that. You just must look into each article and make sure it is UK-based and actually

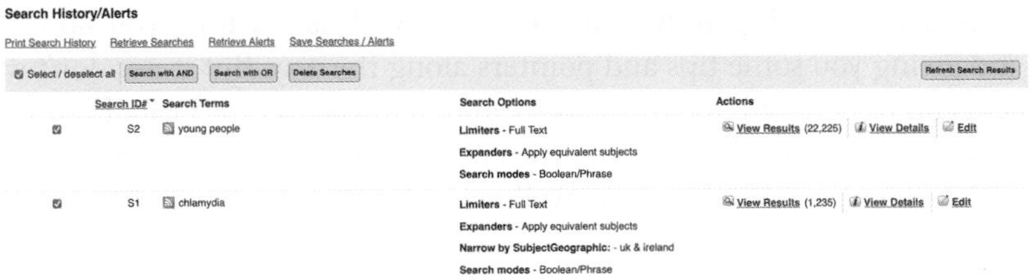

Fig. 4.3 CINAHL complete. Search.

research that's been done in the UK. It is far better to have UK-based research over other countries because the UK is where you're going to be studying and it is where you will be working. Another little thing I have seen is, if you open an article, it might only show you half an article and it doesn't bring up the full article but if you email it to yourself, it actually emails you the full PDF file or full article. I didn't know that either but that's helpful hopefully. It's really frustrating when you can only see half an article, but you want to look at the whole thing so try emailing it to yourself and see if it opens up and hopefully it works for you.

My next database search advice is on Cochrane library now Cochrane, to be honest, it's supposed to be one of the best places to get your research articles from, but I have to be honest, I do struggle a little bit with Cochrane and finding articles. However, I'm just going to give you a small tip which will hopefully help you out with this. During my research, I was looking up pre-exposure prophylaxis for human immunodeficiency virus (HIV) for my final year at university. And again, I was only coming up with one or two papers on this when I knew there was a lot more out there. But stupidly, it was right there in front of me. There is a 'trials' tab that when you press and that brings up a lot more results and when I pressed this, it brought up 319 papers for me. When you open the article just read the abstracts because everything there is in the abstract and you will be able to judge whether you need that in your assignment or not. Then if it is one that you need you can save the article or print it out and go through it thoroughly.

I do find some things on Cochrane, so I do try and use a variety just to help me find more research.

I hope those little tips are going to help you but the main points to remember in database searching is to keep your keywords narrow, and specific and try using different keywords. If that keyword isn't working, narrow it down as much as you can. Remember to use a wide search and use different types of database searches and use different websites to go on.

WRITING REFLECTIONS FOR ASSIGNMENTS

I thought this was actually a really good one to add here because unless someone tells you what to do and how to do it, how do you know how to write a reflection for an assignment? Hopefully, your university will be teaching you how to do this and giving you some tips and pointers along the way. But if not don't worry I'm here and hopefully I am going to try and help you as best I can. Firstly, with reflections, we do this daily without even realising it. We think about what's gone on in the day, what has gone well, what has gone bad, what we could do better to stop something from happening again or how to keep doing something that we do well. It's just finding ways of putting that into academic work or your professional life.

My first tip for this is to think of it like any other assignment. Just because it's a reflection, doesn't mean you're doing things different. So, the main points: you want to make sure it's got good structure and to help you with this structure for your reflection it's always good to use a reflective cycle. For me, I always used the GIBBS model just because I found it the easiest to follow there was a lot of research out there on it and there was a lot of information on the GIBBS cycle and how to write it, so this is why I used the GIBBS cycle. However, I know a lot of people use the Driscoll model and there are a lot of other reflective cycles out there if you want to use them. Have a little look around and find the best one that suits you and as with any assignment, with the structure, you're going to have a start, a middle, and an end just like the rest. Your introductions, main body, and the conclusion. So, the beginning of it is going to be the 'what happened' this is the descriptive bit, and then your main body is going to be explaining a bit more detail such as why is this relevant, why is this relevant to the Nursing and Midwifery Council (NMC) code of conduct for example, and you're going to go to things like policies and procedures and nice guidelines. Build that evidence up on why it's important and why you've recognised this situation that you're reflecting on as high importance if that makes sense. For example, in one of mine, I wrote about a day when we were extremely short-staffed, we were so short-staffed there were 2 nurses to 29 patients on the ward and it was quite a tough time, to be honest. That was one of my last shifts on a ward so I thought I would use this to reflect on it because it was a really good situation to reflect on because actually, even though it wasn't a great situation to be in especially as a student nurse, it was actually a really good learning experience, and the day went really well despite everything. It had two components to the day so I thought this would be really good to write a critical analysis on and show the good sides and the bad sides, what went bad, what went wrong, what went well. Then come to a conclusion on how I'm going to put that in future practice because that's what your conclusion is all about. So, you've had your beginning 'what's happened' then you've had your main body of 'why this is relevant' and this is why it's important according to the NMC code of conduct and the nursing midwifery council guides and standards and procedures and nice guidelines etc. Then the ending, the conclusion, will be how you're going to then improve your future practice; You're going to be doing this, this and this, you're going to put this in place, and this is going to make you a better nurse as a result. In addition, you can pick anything to be your reflection it doesn't matter it doesn't always have to be a bad thing you can always reflect on something that went well and you think 'wow I really want to reflect on this' and then write about it. And this would be the same structure so what happened and then your main body is going to be all about why this is a good thing and relate it again to the NMC code of conduct the standards procedures policies and nice guidelines and all of your trust guidelines. With guidelines and policies, you are allowed to add anything into your assignments that are publicly available to everyone. You are not allowed to add any confidential ones that you cannot access through an online search. Each one must be public to the public domain to be able to use them or you will be pulled up for sharing confidential information and breaching your professional code of conduct. Basically, if you can search online for this at home and it comes up, you can use it. Also, if you're writing about a situation that went well, you want to talk about how you can maintain this for future practice. It's not about improving and changing practices as such. It's more about saying 'okay how do I keep going and what steps am I going to put in place to make sure that this happens again and again, so that I continue to build and improve for other patients in my future practice'.

Now, we will move on to referencing, so I know when I was at university there were a lot of torn things about referencing a reflection. Because it is your own personal experiences but we were always told we have to reference and that's where your main body bit comes into play. Because you're going to be referencing the NMC code, you're going to be referencing the government, you're going to be referencing National Health Service (NHS) England, you're going to be referencing Public Health England, you're going to be referencing the nice guidelines and policies and procedures and hospital trusts. So, yes you can put references in there and not only that, however, you're feeling as a student nurse there's someone who has probably written that somewhere in an article. You can just have a search, get onto your library, and literally just put in a few key words to bring something up, such as student nurse, staff shortages, and student nurse feelings. You will find someone has written an article somewhere like that. Some good online resources for this are places such as Nursing Times, for example, is a good one, Best in Practice Nursing, the Elsevier website as well, nurses.co.uk is another great resource as they share lots of blogs and vlogs from students as well. The Royal College of Nursing Information (RCNi) or Royal College of Nursing (RCN) student network – they do a lot of good articles as well from students. So, use these and put that into your explanations and back that up with your references and say 'okay, well, this is how other people feel as well and it isn't just me. This is how this person felt in this article'. It's quite easy to reference, you just need to get your head around it and put it in and get used to it. It is hard to start with but once you get your head around it, you'll think differently about it, and you'll really get into it…I hope. So, for mine with my staff shortages, I felt nervous about it. I didn't know what to expect, I thought more was going to be expected of me because I was a student nurse and there was a short staffage and I had to be thrown in at the deep end kind of thing. So, I looked around that to see if anyone else had felt this and had the sort of same experiences and who had written an article about it. I found that there were articles about it, so I threw those in there and I just backed up what I was saying to say 'okay I'm not the only person out there that this has happened to because in this article this student explains this too and it's a common thing out there' and then you go into your main body about okay why is this important? So this is important because the NMC says as a student nurse you should not be counted in the numbers, so you shouldn't be used and abused when it's short staffed for example. However, on the other side, if you're confident and competent to do so you *can* help and you can do those things to help. It's weighing it up so that's your pro and that's your con and that's critical analysis in a way. That gave me my overall conclusion because okay even though you're not supposed to be counted in numbers according to the NMC and you're supposed to be supernumerary and learning and things like that. However, on the flip side it says as long as you're competent and confident to do so and your mentor's happy with it and you've got the supervision (they're still supervising from afar) then you are safe to do whatever (well, not whatever you want) but whatever you're trained to do, you can do. In my situation, I felt confident to go out there to help. I was able to take on my own patients to manage it myself with the supervision of my mentor from afar, so I still had that mentor there in the next bay. It turned out well and it turned out like a good day because I'd focused on my autonomy. I had built on the skills that I *could* do, and it just turned out to be, in conclusion, a fantastic shift because of what I had learned.

So, for my conclusion going forward, I would put in 'going forwards I can use all of these skills as a newly qualified nurse, and I know that I've got the autonomy now because I had the confidence to do that and take my own patience and caseload'. I put little bits from what I'd learned from that day and how I would use that as a newly qualified nurse going out there into practice and it just tied in really nicely and it flowed nicely like that so I'm hoping that these tips are going to make yours flow like that.

Just some little basic rules around writing your reflections for an assignment; it's important that you keep it confidential so do not mention the trust or hospital names that you worked in or were on placements in. Do not mention any names in your assignment, literally keep it as minimal as possible because you don't want to break confidentiality and fail as a result. For example, the ward that I worked on was an orthopaedic ward, you can say 'I worked on an orthopaedic ward' but you can't say the name of the hospital, the ward number or the specific trust or anything like that. You cannot add the names of my mentors either. I literally just said 'I was working on an orthopaedic ward and my mentor' and that was it. I didn't use any names, any trust names anything like that. This is the same actually when on social media, you should never tell anyone the location of where you work and that's purely to maintain confidentiality. Because no one can pinpoint where you're talking about or what patients you're talking about or what colleagues you're talking about. You'll see from my social media section more on this and just how important this is.

So, this is just a massive tip, just do not put any names in your assignments. The only time you can reference a name, or a trust is if you're digging out a policy or procedure for a particular trust and then you can put 'in Manchester NHS Trust, they've got a lot of really good policies and guidelines' and 'NHS

Manchester Policy 2018 says this, this and this'. Then you can use it then but if you're talking about your own personal experience, you cannot tell anybody the trust you're working at or anything because it's confidential.

The next thing you need to look at is the next rule; we were always told that for your reflection you can use I, so you can be in first person for the beginning of your reflection because you're talking about yourself and your own experiences. That's okay to do that but then as you write your main body you will go into the third person. I was using the NMC code and things like that to talk about my experiences and then in the conclusion, I switched back to first person. However, that is how our university wanted this structured so, please before you do anything, check with your university's assignment brief guidelines and it should tell you quite clearly what you should be doing and which person to write this in.

To get those extra marks for your reflection assignment, I would advise going a lot more in depth. So, you're not just saying okay this happened and this happened. You're explaining 'why that's important', you're explaining 'how did that make you feel,' you're explaining 'why did you feel that way'. You're going to always be asking yourself 'okay why is that or why am I saying this' or 'why do I feel like this', and you'll keep asking and you'll keep digging to unravel the layers of what's happening. A bit like an onion, you're unravelling all the layers of you and your assignment and you're explaining a little bit more but not only that, you want to add all the critical analysis like we've spoken about already.

And then lastly, again, good references! You want to show your wider reading because wider reading means more points and points mean prizes haha. So, yes good references, good quality references. Make sure you get the research to back it up and don't just put google.com in your references because you're not going to get anywhere with that. In fact, you'll probably get deducted points for writing that so please use good-quality references. You want to use things like research papers, articles, journals, government guidelines, official documents and of course, the NMC has to be in there as well - all the good stuff. It's just about using those good, quality references well in your assignment to get those points and show wider reading.

And lastly, please don't overthink it, please don't panic about it so much, make this easy for yourself rather than harder for yourself. You CAN do this.

FUN FACT

Did you know nurses walk on average between 4 and 5 miles per each 12-hour shift? (Travel Nursing, 2015)

References

CASP. (2022). *Critical Appraisal Skills Programme*. Retrieved from https://casp-uk.net. Accessed 19 May 2022.

CINAHL Complete. (2022a). *EBSCO host [online]*. Retrieved from https://web.p.ebscohost.com/ehost/resultsadvanced?vid=1&sid=369d546a-4463-4b89-959e-a6acacdbe150%40redis&bdata=JmRiPWNjbSZicXVlcnk9JmNsaTA9RlQmY2x2MD1ZJnR5cGU9MSZzZWFyY2hNb2RlPVN0YW5kYXJkJnNpdGU9ZWhvc3QtbGl2ZQ%3d%3d. Accessed 21 May 2022.

CINAHL Complete. (2022b). *EBSCO host [online]*. Retrieved from https://web.p.ebscohost.com/ehost/resultsadvanced?vid=3&sid=b61bcca6-14e9-47d7-b278-6ede623e130a%40redis&bquery=young±people&bdata=JmRiPW5sYWJrJmRiPW5sZWJrJmRsaTA9TkwmZGx2MD1ZJmRsZDA9bmxhYmsmdHlwZT0xJnNlYXJj-aE1vZGU9U3RhbmRhcmQmc2l0ZT1laG9zdC1saXZl%3d. Accessed 21 May 2022.

Lehane, E., Leahy-Warren, P., O'Riordan, C., Savage, E., Drennan, J., O'Tuathaigh, C., et al. (2019). Evidence-based practice education for healthcare professions: an expert view. *BMJ Evidence-based Medicine*, 24(3), 103–108. doi: http://dx.doi.org/10.1136/bmjebm-2018-111019. In this issue.

Nottingham University. (n.d.). *Studying Effectively: Types of writer*. Available at: https://www.nottingham.ac.uk/studyingeffectively/writing/writer/types.aspx. Accessed 30/12/2022.

The University of Nottingham. (2014). *An academic support handbook for students*. Retrieved from https://www.nottingham.ac.uk/studentservices/documents/planning-and-preparing-to-write-assignments.pdf. Accessed 23 June 2021.

Travel Nursing. (2015). *The 4 mile shift: why nurses walk so much*. Retrieved from https://www.travelnursing.com/news/features-and-profiles/the-4-mile-shift-how-far-do-nurses-walk/. Accessed 16 May 2022.

CHAPTER 5

Poster Presentations! 'HELP!'

Public speaking is one thing I really needed to work on, this includes poster presentations. I dreaded the thought of speaking in public. So, when the bombshell was dropped that we would do weekly poster presentations in front of the whole class – I began to sweat.

Although I think it is safe to say, most of us in that classroom began to sweat. However, we had to do weekly presentations to get us practicing and prepared for the real deal: Our marked presentation. And this really helped me get used to presenting in front of people and by the time the big day came, I wasn't as nervous. I will never forget the first conference I spoke at; I was so nervous on the day, and someone said to me just before 'think of it as, it's not about you, it's about sharing your story and helping others'. This really helped me to focus on the reason I was doing something like that, which helped greatly! Another thing I had learnt was to remind yourself when you have been to a talk or presentation, did you really care about the person themselves? Were you passing judgement on them? The answer is probably no because realistically people don't sit there judging you. So why would anyone sit there and do this to you? So be kind to yourself, it's going to be ok. I know this will be very different at university and being graded on a presentation because you want to do well. But the same applies to that, no one wants you to fail, and everyone in that room wants you to do well and pass. So just do your best ☺

The best piece of advice I can give here is:

- To calm your nerves on the day, look around the room and start naming things silently in your head, table, chair, desk, pen, poster, windows etc.
- Use breathing techniques to help regulate your breath
- For the presentation: Write flashcards with bullet points to keep you on track rather than a long-winded script
- Practice, practice, and practice before the big day
- Ask your university if there are any opportunities for you to do talks to other classes or any new first-year students that are starting. This really helped me so much with my public speaking skills – push through those fears
- Get your friend, family, partner or even your pet to sit down and listen to your presentation. Keep going over it with them and this will help on the main day
- Don't forget to time your presentation when you practice – presentations are often timed, and you do not want to go over your time limit

- The examiner is not looking at how you look or appear, they want to know that you know what you're talking about. The more you practice and know your stuff the better – So, don't worry about being nervous, this is natural to most people – You are human and not a robot at the end of the day
- If you are using a PowerPoint presentation, keep it minimal. Do not overload your PowerPoint with too much information. You just want short basic queues to remind you what to talk about next. Sometimes this is nice to put in a powerful image relevant to what you're talking about too

Where to Begin?

1. Read your assignment brief and narrow it down
2. Use the assignment brief/guide and marking criteria to set your structure of the presentation
3. How can you make it visual? What can you add to the poster to make it stand out?
4. What information can you deliver during your presentation that will complement this?
5. Decide what is the best software or paper to use for your poster: We used PowerPoint presentation for ours which worked well
6. If using computer software, make sure you use a very plain background so that people can read off the screen. Coloured backgrounds don't always work well
7. Plan how many slides you need for how many minutes you have: I had one slide for every minute, which kept it simple

What Makes a Good Poster?

- Information should be readable
- Use shorter words to gain interest
- Keep it to the point and clear
- Use bullet points, numbers, and headlines can make it easier to read
- Use of graphics and colour to make it interesting
- Clear layout
- Includes acknowledgements/references throughout and a reference list at the end

FUN FACT

Did you know the first nursing school was opened in India in 250 BCE, and only men could apply! (Christensen, 2017)

Reference

Christensen, M. (2017). Men in nursing: The early years. *Journal of Nursing Education and Practice, 7*(5). https://doi.org/10.5430/jnep.v7n5p94. Accessed 10 May 2022.

CHAPTER 6

Level 4 to 7 Marking Criteria and Critically Analysing

For the first year, your assignments and exams are marked at a level 4 marking criteria. In the second year, it goes up to level 5 and in the third year to level 6. Some students find the jump from level 4 to level 5 quite hard. First year, seems like such a breeze when I look back now. Please don't be disheartened if your results drop in second year a little bit – this happened to me. During the first year I got average grades between 80% and 90% but in second year they dropped between 60% and 75% which was a little bit soul-destroying to me. However, this was because the level had gone up and I hadn't raised my writing level up with it. Here are my top tips for surviving that jump:

- Critically analyse every paragraph if you can.
- Ensure your references are evidence-based practice and a variety of different pieces of research to back your evidence up. The more (good) references you have – this shows your wider reading. Evidence-based practice: research papers, articles, academic work.

At level 4, you are just describing things, and explaining things. At level 5 you want to be critically analysing everything and backing up what you are saying with evidence-based practice. Finding good quality research to back up what you're saying as well.

What Is Critically Analysing?

This is far simpler than you think! A fantastic lecturer explained it like this; think of it as buying a mobile phone. You do not know which one to choose from. First, you want to know which model to have, then which colour to have, what camera features are the best on which phone, how much memory do you want etc. The pros and cons of each one. Then once you have all your facts about each phone model, you will come to a conclusion on which one to buy based on your research. You have just critically appraised! Now you just have to apply this to whatever your assignment is about.

For another example, in one assignment that I did on wound management, I used all the evidence to show which types of dressings work for this wound and which ones didn't work, but then I rationalised which dressing to use by the research on each dressing, but also costing too. So once, I had found my dressing type (which was a plain Mepore dressing) I then weighed up the cost of the dressings, as there was more than one standard dressing for this wound. So, I went with the cheapest, best available product for my patient. This is what you do to critically analyse something in an assignment and the more you can do the better.

Academic Skills, Assessment and Academic Integrity – By Ann-Marie Dodson

Congratulations whatever you have been doing got you a university place. Well done. However, now is the time that you consider *how* you study, take notes, read etcetera and consider what your strengths and weaknesses are in relation to an academic course? Being a registered nurse today involves many employability skills gained from the academic study and the professional training that you will be undertaking in university and placement. Both University and placement are incredibly intertwined. You need to ensure your skill set and ability is evenly balanced. You can do this by taking time to plan, prepare and prioritise and enjoy your journey to becoming a nurse.

There are many routes into nursing today from the traditional A-levels, Access to Higher Education, NVQs (National Vocational Qualifications), Baccalaureates, Foundation degrees and Transition to Nursing Courses. Some of you will be studying Apprentice Nursing or a degree at the master's level. This chapter is based on over 40 years experience of working clinically and 30 years in university teaching post-registration and pre-qualifying students. Although each University is slightly different, the over-arching principles of studying and assessments will be discussed. It is recommended that you do your own research on your specific chosen University and course. You also need to be clear about what 'nursing' is and how demanding a university course in nursing is. Be clear about your expectations and how good your academic and writing skills are, or not. It's about self-awareness as universities have various courses to help, but it takes the student to recognise that they have some limitations.

So, do your homework. Review all the websites and do your research and mindset as it's a 3-year commitment if you are choosing a BSc, possibly four if a master's or, a dual award. Speak to family and friends. Reach out to other student nurses on Facebook, Twitter or Instagram. Go to Open days and speak to staff and students.

GETTING STARTED WITH YOUR ACADEMIA

There are students that see the academic part of the course as separate from the clinical part of the course. They can really flourish and achieve highly in clinical practice as they are gifted practically with great interpersonal and communication skills. However, you also need the academic skills to be able to reach your goals. Clinical practice and academia are two sides of the same coin which you need to appreciate. You cannot be a registered Nurse without passing all parts of your course. Neglect one part at your peril. So, you need to be honest with yourself, as well as with your personal tutor and academic assessor. They will respect you more and be more able to guide and support you. Really address your strengths and limitations to studying and academic writing. They can then guide and support you appropriately. Take stock now. Developing good self-awareness at the start of your studies will enable you to access the wealth of resources and extra-curricular short courses that will be available. These lessons will apply throughout your academic and professional life at whatever level you are studying. Achieving the status of a nurse is only the start of your academic life, as a tenet of nursing and registration with the NMC (Nursing and Midwifery Council, 2019) is that we must re-validate every 3 years and prove that we have kept learning, reflecting, and developing. Nursing is a life-long journey of learning. Knowledge is constantly expanding and practice evolving and changing, and we must develop alongside that to be safe and competent practitioners.

At course induction, and the start of each new academic year there will be study and library skills sessions. It is advised that you attend these even if you feel skilled already as you may get a surprise, or at least reinforce your previous learning. For example, the referencing system can differ, and expectations are different to those you may have experienced previously. There again, you may have been working and out of study for some years. This can impact your confidence but remember all the life skills that you gained will prove useful.

In addition to the course, year, and module inductions, academic skills workshops outside the main course are offered throughout the year by university staff that are dedicated to supporting students with academic and writing skills. Students with good grades also seek to support to improve their work further. There are also specialist tutors to help those with neurodiversity, particularly dyslexia. Teachers of 'English as a foreign Language' are often available but if you feel your written English could be a challenge it may be worth enrolling on a functional skills course, or classes at a local language centre or, College of further education. Other University and Faculty staff will also advertise and share their expertise such as the library staff. They offer one-to-one, group tutorials or workshops on referencing and literature searching. The IT departments often have experts in learning technology and offer the same format as the library staff in respect of computer skills such as creating and storing word documents, to generating power-points and spreadsheets. Don't forget the wealth of information and tutorials on the web such as YouTube videos and Ted talks which are invaluable.

No one will make you do anything. You are an adult learner. You need to take responsibility. The best students are those who can learn how to learn, are curious and self-directed. I suggest that you do not want to be finding out your weaknesses at the end of the first year when you are having to deal with several re-submissions, often at the same time, which is extremely stressful. Such a situation can impact your progression within the course and on occasion lead to withdrawal from the course. Hindsight is a wonderful thing but let's avoid this situation by putting in some thought and effort at the start. Better still, before you start!

The first year of most courses and certainly the first semester or term is about finding your feet. This involves learning about yourself, the University, the Faculty and most importantly the course. You will be making new friends and getting to know the staff. You need to know who the course and module leads are, as well as becoming familiar with the rules, regulations, policies and procedures.

This same learning and familiarity will apply to the practice area. This is a time of huge change and transition for you. You will feel overwhelmed with all the information you will be given. It can be very stressful if you have not prepared properly and done some problem-solving in advance. It could spoil your experience. Don't let this happen. This first year as I describe it, is a 'levelling up' time, as the entry gate is wide, as is the experience of all the students. It is a time when staff can assess your capabilities, strengths, and weaknesses. It is a 'diagnostic' of sorts and is not only about academic staff assessing you in so many ways, but also you are hopefully reflecting and making some judgements about yourself. This may require you to make some adjustments or, new plans.

WHY IS ACADEMIA SO IMPORTANT?

Many students tell me that they came into nursing as they are practical people. Many did not have positive experiences at school and that baggage follows us. Many can be in a state of anxiety. Many initially think to themselves all will be ok as their clinical reports are good, and this is where they excel. However, they still need to be able to pass their academic assessments.

The skills you learn in academia are equally as important as the clinical ones. You will need to be able to write and communicate effectively in English. This is an NMC requirement. The NMC Code (2018a) has a specific section which mentions the standard required of a registered nurse. There are some trained nurses that have been struck off from the register because they could not meet this standard. It can lead to mistakes in practice and poor and unsafe practices. Registration is a separate issue but to successfully complete the degree and your studies, you will need to pass ALL your modules. The various forms of assessment and criteria will be discussed in more depth shortly.

You need to be able to write and read effectively as you will be dealing with lots of information in the clinical area. This can range from patient care pathways, treatment plans, referral letters and charting results. You will be writing in the patient's notes and discussing care with the medical staff and multi-disciplinary team. You need to be accurate. A mistake can lead to a communication error or even serious harm. Spelling a word wrongly can have consequences and there will be many new medical and clinical words and phrases to master. You will learn a new vocabulary and culture. With time you will develop your learning and competence alongside strategies that work for you. You will always be supervised. You will be developing and delivering teaching sessions throughout your studies and training, as well as writing policies and reports (mostly later in your career but it depends on the assessment tasks that you will be set by your module leaders).

All care must be based on evidence and research-based literature (NMC, 2018b). We will look at this later in the chapter, but all assessments need to show that you have read widely and that you are applying this learning in your academic work and clinically. On occasion, a student must write a statement after an incident in practice or, even give evidence in court although rarer. Therefore, the ability to write coherently is crucially important. However, you can be supported by the University and the hospital trust. The Student's Union can also help or even the Trade Unions, such as the RCN (Royal College of Nursing).

I have known a few students rationalise poor performance by saying that they only need to 'pass' the module. If you are trying your best that is one thing and staff will try and assist, but if you are repeatedly being referred in a module you need to question, why is this happening, and can I do anything about it? Put yourself in a patient's shoes for an instant. They will expect you to be knowledgeable and competent as a registrant.

WHAT DO I NEED TO BUY?

I'm a pragmatist. Keep your spending as low as possible. With all the excitement you can get carried away. You are a student and although Claire has 'hacks' to help, you will have a limited income.

Your biggest purchase is the most important, and that is a laptop or computer. Get advice from a computer shop or the Faculty IT department as there can be an incompatibility between operating systems. You might then have to convert documents which add to the stress and pressure if your skills are underdeveloped. Using your mobile phone is not the answer as sometimes timetables and assessment feedback cannot be seen due to data issues.

- A laptop that is light and portable and will see you through your course. It is the best investment you can make and there are student discounts and deals. Big retailers and the Faculty IT can advise. An external hard drive may be useful so you can back up your work. Ensure that you have reliable 'connectivity'. A laptop can go in and out of the university with you and will often be useful in class for taking notes or following a lecture in real time.
- Review your broad-band-internet provision as there will be some blended learning in every university course. You may need a 'dongle'. I have sometimes had to find a café or pub to be able to get access but there are the noise and confidentiality aspects to consider. So, think about what you

would do if you had no access or your computer breaks. This is vital if you are writing an assessment or uploading work to the university. Always plan, prepare, and have plans A and B.

- Pen, pencils, rubber, paper, sticky notelets, flashcards and notebooks are all useful.
- A rucksack (take care of your back as you are relying on it for your living. Nursing involves manual handling and moving patients and very long hours of standing).
- You can use spelling and grammar checkers on your computer. But there are applications on many phones that you can install a calculator, dictionary, and thesaurus.
- Prospective students ask what books should I buy? Most courses will have online book lists for the course and every module. University libraries not only hold hard copies of books and journals but most of the key stock is available electronically. It is mostly journals that you will be referring to for your assessments which will be based on the evidenced-base and research literature.

If I was to buy a book, I would choose an Anatomy and Physiology text recommended by the staff. This will last you for many years as it is not likely to become outdated. A pharmacology book related to nursing would also be an investment. After that, it's your choice but for Christmas and birthdays, you can ask always to ask for book vouchers. At the start of the academic year, especially at university induction, publishers often offer discounts. Banks and Unions will also offer such incentives and of course, you can always buy second-hand from the various websites.

Now We Have Covered the Generalities, Let's Think About the Specifics

When designing a course and module, academics must consider the standards and proficiencies laid down by the professional body (NMC, 2018c). In addition, all Higher Education institutions are required to adhere to the standards set by the QAA (Quality Assurance Agency) which provides data to the OFS (Office for Students). In addition, some courses are inspected by Ofsted (the Office for Standards and Education, children's services, and skills) as well as HEE (Health Education England). There can be variations across the UK. All courses are therefore designed to meet specific standards. They are 'validated' for a set period before a review. They are constantly monitored through internal and external quality assurance processes. You will be asked for feedback and to evaluate every aspect of your course at set times. There are External Examiners who work in other Universities who review your work after it has been marked and moderated within the home institution. This ensures that your education is fit for purpose and that you achieve the set standard for achieving a degree as it needs to be consistent and comparable within universities and courses.

There are some that think a nursing degree may be an easier option than some other types of degree that may be available in health care, but you will find this is not the case.

When designing a course, it is important that the chosen assessment method aligns or matches the content (subject material) of the module and the learning objectives (the things you should be able to do after undertaking the module and having learnt the content). The academics will also ensure that the assessment methods vary, so it would not be possible for a nursing course in the UK to be based solely on exams as many years ago. This is a good thing as some students excel at exams and others do not. Having a mix of methods will ensure that you can work to your strengths. Do you know what they are?

EXAMS: NUMERACY

All student nurses will have numeracy exams every year. These must be passed on to progress through the course. This is my weak area, but I have strategies for dealing with it. There are electronic systems for undertaking these exams such as 'safe-medicate'. You will be told what the pass rate is each year and will have the opportunity to practice. There is generally one resit opportunity. This is because this skill is crucial to patient safety. Although the university has a pass rate (usually 40% for undergraduate work from levels 4 to 6 and master's level at 50%) you should be aiming for 100%. Any error in practice in the real world could cause harm. It could also cause death. Drug calculation and administration are the fundamental roles of the nurse.

The university will help you to prepare through teaching, tutorials and quizzes. There are maths tutors for those that need extra help as you may have a learning difficulty like dyscalculia. You can apply to the student disability service for testing if you suspect this and any student with a learning difficulty or health condition, can be assessed and often be granted a support summary. This can outline reasonable adjustments such as extra time. However, this would not be possible in a health care setting in real time, to give someone extra time to complete a drug round. Every student is measured against the NMC proficiencies, which are really a set of skills. Drug calculation and administration are two of them. You may be able to take your exam at home or, more likely in university, and often in an exam or assessment centre.

If you are one of those that becomes a bag of nerves when exams are mentioned, you need to start addressing your fear. The university will offer sessions on preparing for exams, tacking exam nerves, meditation techniques and developing strategies for example. Preparing is key, as that will give you confidence. For example, do you know where the exam will be held? Do a dummy run so that you can time your journey, know the route and the room. Can you park if you are driving? Do have your breakfast. Take some water. You do not want to get up late and be all flustered. Depending on the time you arrive, if you are late for an exam, you may be allowed to enter, but you will have less time to complete it. You will be told if you need a calculator. Do not cheat. You will be expected to adhere to the NMC Code (2018d) which requires nurses to be honest and have integrity. There is usually a couple of minutes reading time. Don't skip this. Read the instructions carefully. Make sure you answer all the parts that you are required to do and in the set time. I would suggest working methodically as if you skip back and forth you may miss a section. Practice typing at speed, and your handwriting, in case you must revert to paper.

If you are ill and this is going to impair your performance, let the staff know that you will not be attending and why. Follow the university procedure for such eventualities. If you attempt the assessment, you are stating that you are 'fit to sit'. If you are not successful, and later claim that you were unwell, you may find that you are not allowed to retrieve that attempt. Every decision that you make, or don't make has consequences.

The usual reason students are unsuccessful in exams (referred or failed) is inadequate preparation. You must revise. Exams are based on knowledge recall. They have advantages as they are relatively quick to mark, and we can assess all aspects of a taught module and your knowledge and understanding. The downside of having just crammed the night before unless you have got an excellent short-term memory, and can you regurgitate material, is that cramming does not push and store material in the deeper memory. So, I could argue that you have not learnt it. Learning is said to be a permanent change and you should be able to recall it many years later as a nurse.

If you are highly anxious, then you will not learn effectively as it impairs memory. So, seek help early and even consider seeing a psychologist, getting hypnotherapy, or using a private tutor to help you. The important thing is to address your fears. You can do it, especially if you focus on your long-term goal of being a nurse.

So, What Other Exams Will I Have to Take?
MCQS AND SHORT ANSWER QUESTIONS

There will be most likely another exam every year to test your knowledge and recall related to a clinical module usually. This may contain elements of pharmacology and physiology.

Such exams usually take the form of a mix of multiple-choice questions (MCQs) and short answer questions. I would advise you to always keep up your skill of writing with a pen and paper in case there is a technical problem on the day. It will be more likely that you will be using a keyboard. If you need an adapted one, ensure that the module leads know this well in advance. But if you are like me and finger type, you will be slower than those that can speed type. So, don't run out of time. That said, consider your answers carefully. Some advice is going with your gut, and give your first answer for MCQs, but also take a minute to think about the question. What is the examiner asking? Make sure that you understand the question and the choices given. Some of this is common sense, but I will often use a process of elimination of what I think the wrong response is and work through the responses logically using 'deductive reasoning'. You will be given reading time and don't be tempted to start answering until you have read the instructions and have the measure of what questions the paper contains.

On occasion, there are 'Open book' exams where you can pre-prepare by being given a topic or overview of a question or case and can utilise references from material that you have read.

EXAMS: OSCEs

There may be an OSCE (objective structured clinical assessment). This can be used to measure clinical knowledge and skills related to practice and the professional component of the course. Again, every university is different. If they are included in your course you will be well briefed and prepared. You will be given the opportunity to practice. Many Faculties have 'learning spaces' or clinical rooms where students can practice informally. There will be equipment and procedures to use and follow. The OSCE may involve using simulation on a mannikin or a member of staff. This is much better than the trial-and-error learning that I did in my training often undertaking a skill in real time for the very first time on a patient. Practising in a safe environment at university or, in a clinical placement and simulating, or role-playing, is much better than making an error with a patient. It means that you will feel much more confident and in control when you do it for the first time with a real person.

It is of course nerve-wracking, but examiners take this into account. Be systematic. Deep breath and keep calm. Don't forget to introduce yourself, adhere to infection control procedures, consider the environment and comfort of the patient. To gain consent, document and most importantly 'communicate' with your patient. Learn the steps that they have taught you and be safe. Safety is paramount in nursing. Up to 300 hours of the 2300 hours of clinical practice required to be a nurse can be undertaken through some form of simulation.

ACADEMIC ASSESSMENTS

These come in many forms from traditional written essays, literature reviews, dissertations, care plans, PowerPoint presentations to reports. Each one is a different task. All will require you to write (and sometimes speak) effectively in English. The skills of structuring your work logically, spelling and grammar are integral and transferrable. You will also need to support your work with appropriate quality sources from the literature. Your opinion is valued but not all work is based on your opinion and needs to be supported with evidence and research. Being able to apply your reading is paramount. Reading for your degree is fundamental. You need to put the time and work in. There are no easy or quick fixes. The more you read the more you will learn and understand. You will notice the academic style of the Author and how they reference what sources they use, and your style will develop consequently.

KEY POINTS

When starting off with any assessment consider when is it due to be submitted and how? Note the date and time of submission in your diary and phone. When are the re-submissions attempts? Plan those into your diary or calendar also just in case. There are also study planners from your faculty such as the library or centres that deal with 'academic skills for success' and the web (you can refer to TED talks, podcasts, and YouTube). There are also plenty of study skills guides and books. We have a few in our reference list. This will all be covered at induction when you start University.

What you must not do, is leave your academic work to the last minute. It is easy to forget about assignments if you are on placement and tired. Work back from the deadline. Tutorials are not usually offered the week before hand-in as University staff do not want to be reinforcing bad habits as you are expected to plan. That said, recognise when you are in difficulty and seek help and guidance as early as you can.

Do attend your module launch, and any session launching the assessment. Although this will be in written format and often recorded, it is much better to hear it live. Don't be afraid to ask questions for clarification. If you don't understand a point, there will be others in your group that will be glad that you asked. Each assessment type will have been validated when the course was originally written. Each year slight changes may be made but the assessment itself will be independently internally reviewed by the module team and externally reviewed by the 'External Examiner'.

The nursing course itself will have been co-produced by placement staff as well as academics. Current students and ex-students are also an important part of curriculum development, as are 'experts by experience'. So, the assessment should be as well developed and clear as possible. That said some students will feel that they don't understand the assessment and what they need to do. This is normal.

So, first, don't panic. Take things a step at a time. Print off the assessment brief if you can, as well as the assessment criteria, and any guidelines. If you follow these then you are halfway to passing. What are the learning outcomes? What skills are required? What is the objective of the assessment? Each assessment is designed to measure the learning in that module. It is launched at the start or, near to the start, but academics will keep referring to it and ensure as best as they can that there is an understanding well before the hand-in date. You need to be patient as with anything in life you need to take your time and keep re-reading the brief. Discuss it with your peers and attend any tutorials.

A useful tip is to use a highlighter pen and *underline* the key words. Develop a plan and don't expect to write your assignment as soon as it is given. Do not try and pass work off that seems similar from a previous course. There is something called self-plagiarism. This is not allowed. Once you understand the task you need to start reading. You will have been given a course and module reading list. Academics may have given you specific reading to do with their session. You can do your own search for material. Try and use the most contemporary material that you can. Some more dated material can be acceptable if it is what is described as 'seminal' for instance, the first time a theory was written about. Remember that much literature that nursing refers to is not unique to the profession as we use knowledge from medicine, pharmacology, sociology and physiology for example. The skill is to apply this to our practice. Your work will need constant editing and refining until it is of a quality to submit it. Be patient. Take a break from it. Read it aloud. Use your spell and grammar checker. Ensure that your referencing meets the requirement of your faculty. What you used previously at your college or school may not use the same system. Again, there are referencing guides that the staff will guide you to, and they are often on the library site also. It is possible and sometimes acceptable to use programmes or apps but learn how to do it yourself first. Like any skill, you need to understand it and practice it. Poor referencing won't fail your assignment but may impact the quality and mark awarded. It is a fundamental academic skill. You will need to be able to reference when you are a qualified nurse when developing policies and procedures. You will be expected to support or back up your points and utilise what you have read and learnt. If you haven't read widely and used varied and credible sources this will have an impact on the quality of your work and the grade. Don't forget to use government sources such as the DHSC (Department of Health and Social Care), bodies such as the King's Fund, ONS (Office for National Statistics), WHO (World Health Organization) as well as government websites.

TAKING NOTES

You will feel you want to write everything down. Is this feasible? For some people, it helps to keep focus, but you can get stressed and lost if you are trying to write down 'verbatim'. You need to maintain your skills in handwriting as it will be needed in practice or in if unable to use a digital device. It needs to be legible. Some students are allowed to use voice recorders if they need 'reasonable adjustments' under the Equality Act (2010). Some sessions will be recorded but not all. If you are recording you do need to ask permission from the teacher and

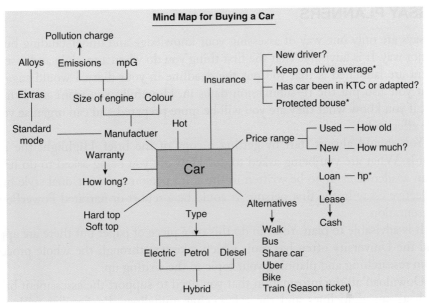

Fig. 6.1 Photo of a mind map on paper. (Photo by Ann-Marie Dodson.)

remember that the content of the lesson can be sensitive, involve other students and is confidential.

So how do you take notes effectively? You need to be able to listen effectively but extract the main points. You can do this in a notebook by just listening or, even better if you use a mind-mapping technique (Fig. 6.1).

There are apps to help with this such as 'Mind-Genius'.

The concept is that using text bubbles with a central word or concept (the main topic) in the middle of the page but work outwards. The resulting diagram is easy to look at. Images or drawings can work well for some. It organises your thoughts. You can plan an assignment like this. There is research to show that the higher-grade students do well using this technique. It saves time and makes revision easier. Some students go on later that day to revise these jottings or notes and write them up. It would be a better use of time to read around the topic, but we all work and learn differently.

Developing flashcards are useful as they allow you to focus down to the main points, use colours or drawings and are a useful 'aide-memoire' when revising. Making notes from one lecture and never doing any more work will not get you that degree. The information needs to be driven into long-term memory and be retrievable and applied in your essays and in the care of patients.

Some students find 'sticky notes' invaluable for noting key points and have them dotted around the house, on the fridge, the toilet door and some even have their walls plastered in them. It's whatever works for you and if your family tolerate it. A good test of whether you have learnt something is that you can teach it.

ESSAY PLANNERS

Essays are only one way of assessing your knowledge and understanding but a major way. It is advisable that the first thing you do when a module and assessment are launched is that you put the deadline in your diary. I would suggest that you also put the re-submission dates in. Hopefully, you won't need them but if you know what they are you will be more prepared and can organise your life effectively.

You should always start by getting a copy of the brief. Highlight the key words. What are you being asked to do? How are you being asked to do it? Is it an academic essay to be written in the third person or impersonal style or, a reflective essay in the first person? It could be a report or narrated PowerPoint presentation.

It is advisable to plan. You can do this on a piece of paper but there are apps, and the University often has tools which take you through the whole process from researching and planning your topic to the writing up.

Download all the information that you need to support the assessment brief such as any guidelines and the referencing guidelines. Be familiar with the assessment and or marking criteria.

READING

It may seem impertinent to talk about reading as you clearly can if you got into university, but if you can improve your skill and speed, you will find academia much easy.

- Before you start University it would be sensible to get your eyes tested. Upgrade your glasses if you need to. Always have a spare pair.
- Have a study place with good lighting.
- Have a highlighter/pencil to hand
- Use a book stand if possible or make sure you hold the book at arm's length in line with your eyes as you would with a computer screen
- Take breaks and look into the distance regularly to ensure you rest the eyes and allow the eyes to re-accommodate.

Historically across all World cultures, it was the religious groups who were the scholars and later the ruling classes and those described as the intelligentsia. There are many illiterate people across the World even in the UK. Not all children get an education, and our reading ages can vary. We hear this when students are presenting in class with nerves put aside. Some students read fluently and have good comprehension, articulacy and vocabulary. These are all skills that are needed in placement and can be improved like any skill. Confidence and self-belief will develop with time.

Start by reading whenever you can. This can be a paperback for pleasure or a glossy magazine. When researching your chosen topic start with the easier material to get a feel of the subject. At this point, it is acceptable to do a quick internet search on GOOGLE or Wikipedia, but you would never be expected to reference them directly as you need to go on and search for more pertinent, credible, subject-specific and evidence-based material. For instance, if you only read red-label newspapers, the topics and language maybe not be as wide-ranging and intellectually stretching as that in the 'broadsheets' which are content-heavy. When you are reading for university work hopefully you will be noticing the author's academic style, the words they use, how they structure the work, form their arguments, what sources they use and how they reference in the text and the list. Just reading should improve your skills if you are observant and thoughtful.

Most of the reading you will be doing will not necessarily be book-based but articles and sometimes government policies or reports. The principles are the same. You cannot read everything, and you need to start to be discerning as there are so many sources available to you, but in a finite amount of time. Prioritise.

One tip before reading is the get an overview of the content. There may be an abstract or index. Review the introduction and conclusion and the headings, sub-headings, reading the first land last sentences. Is it useful to you? This is a key question This should give you a sense of the work. If not move on. Don't be distracted. This is a discipline that you need to develop.

This technique is useful for revision too as it just helps you revisit concepts, facts, and theories that you have learnt previously and helps commit it to memory. But don't forget you need to be able to retrieve it also.

Sometimes, you may find something that may be relevant to another topic and that's fine, just take a note of it or save it, put it away and move on. Focus on the task in hand. Another key skill.

Diagrams or tables can be useful as they summarise and are information rich. Some learners find the visual cues easier.

So, when you are reading vary the pace, read out loud as often as you can, look out for key words, look for repetition. Is the author suggesting causation and summarising the main points or arguments? This will determine whether you can skim over it and whether it's useful to you.

Reading critically or in more detailed reading is more time-consuming. This requires more skill and commitment. You need a good work environment, and you need to ask yourself some important questions. Is the argument, train of thought or proposition logical? Is it biased and is there evidence to support the content and conclusions drawn?

This detailed reading requires practice like any skill. It will be tiring. Plan your time. Try and read every day. You will get faster. You need time to consider, analyse and reflect. You need to think about the facts, the words and the propositions used. A dictionary and thesaurus are invaluable and are often standard applications on most computers and devices. Looking up words that you don't understand is crucial. I spent a lot of time on one module explaining what a 'rationale' was, as the students couldn't grasp it and therefore couldn't write a care plan as they needed to give a rationale (or justification) for a nursing intervention. Words are as powerful as knowledge and experience.

Take a few moments to consider what you have learnt (Clarke, 2017). Do this after every session and at the end of every day. Maybe write a few bullet points or a synopsis. Consider why it is relevant to your learning? If you have been on placement, maybe it relates to a patient that you looked after. For instance, you have just been taught the Anatomy and Physiology (A&P) of the heart and are reviewing an article on caring for a patient with a heart attack or an MI (myocardial infarction. Relating the theory (concepts and facts) and seeing the application to the care of the patient will help your learning and recall in an exam or, a practical setting.

So, my first experience of university was a long time ago and very different. It was assumed that we had good academic, writing and study skills already and we had no guidance or teaching. My second was in relation to nursing at the certificate level, but no assumptions were made. One technique we were taught is SQ3R.

SO, WHAT IS SQ3R?

SQ3R is a technique that will save you a lot of time if you can master it. It will need practice and discipline. SQR stands for survey, question, question, read, recite, and review.

As a student nurse, you will need to read and assimilate a lot of information quickly and use it. This will be in university and clinically. You start by surveying the document or skim reading. Let your eyes dart about but in a systematic way so that you get a quick idea of the content and structure. When searching for literature for research or literature-based material for your essays, you will need to be critical and use your judgement otherwise you will want to read everything which isn't possible.

You can speed up your reading if you finger point or use your finger to trace the page from left to right. If it's a book think about where you hold it as it saves re-reading if you do this effectively and think about your peripheral vision. Lifting your eyes and looking at the ceiling or into the distance occasionally will stop your eyes from getting tired.

As you read, ask yourself questions such as 'is this relevant?', 'what are the main points?' As you are scanning and skimming you are trying to get the 'gist' of the piece. Then you read it again. This time it's a much more active process and you are actively reading this about considering the complexities of the material and understanding in more depth. When you do this you will relate to previous experience and knowledge. Now you can take notes. Building on pieces of knowledge is what educationalists call 'scaffolding'.

Dividing up a complex task and making it smaller is the best way of working whilst organising you are also prioritising, dividing the complex bigger task into smaller more manageable and understandable pieces of information.

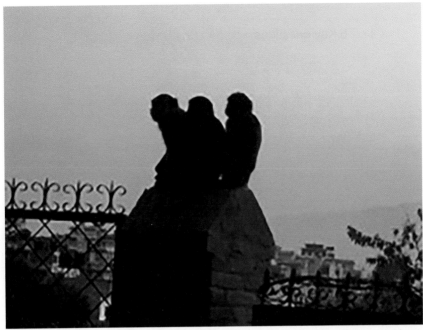

Fig. 6.2 Three wise monkeys at Swayambhunath Temple, Nepal. (Photo by Ann-Marie Dodson.)

The key questions you always need to ask yourself are 'What, who, when and why and how?' The five 'W's and 1 'H' are the tenets of writing and journalism. I always think of the three wise monkeys (Fig. 6.2).

As well as developing your vocabulary which is crucial to be able to develop your literary different levels of understanding and knowledge, it will help you remember and develop your attention span. It is a good habit to develop to reflect on your day and consider what you have learnt and what more you need to explore? The five key questions (Fig. 6.3) will be invaluable whether you are working on an academic assignment or clinically.

Academic Assessments: What Are We Measuring?

So, all the preceding information is the foundation for you to be able to write an effective essay. You need to have understanding of some of the educational terminology. The curriculum is the 'master plan' of all the taught material, clinical skills and experiences that you need to study, to become a registered nurse. There will be differences depending on which course you chose based on the level. For instance, a bachelor's programme as opposed to a master's degree comprise different educational levels, and the amount of content and length differ. All will be validated by the NMC as any course is governed by the University.

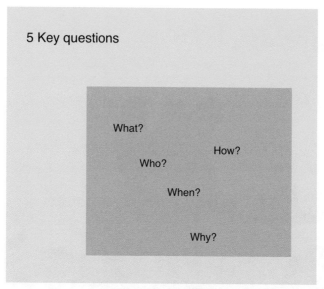

Fig. 6.3   Five key questions.

Over the years the entry gate to university has widened to ensure inclusivity but means that there are a variety of routes into education. This can lead to a difference in educational background and skill set. The first year of any programme is about levelling up and getting to know the University, the Faculty, policies and requirements of the course as well as getting to know staff and make friends.

You will hear the phrase '*learning outcomes*'. These are statements that are written so that we can measure whether our teaching strategies and approaches and your consequent learning. The Learning outcomes should match with the course and module content and should be measurable through the set assessment.

An educational taxonomy by Armstrong (2010) (Fig. 6.4), which was originally developed in 1956. It is a good way to understand the skills that are being measured. Level 4 is a certificate level and is about knowledge and understanding. It's about being able to recall and explain facts. This is the foundational level of your studies. As you progress in your course you will rise the pyramid in terms of the skills and their complexity. More will be demanded by the assessments as you progress through your course.

Your faculty will help you prepare for your studies, but you will only get out of it what you put in and there will be no fun and enjoyment if you are in a constant state of anxiety. Ask for help when you need to. Speak to your peers. Use all the resources available to you and there are many study skills books available. Most of all keep focused but make some time for yourself and embrace the challenge. Keep curious and enjoy. Each day you are nearer to your goal of being a nurse.

As you progress through your course the emphasis will move from remembering, knowledge and understanding. At level 5, the level recognised within

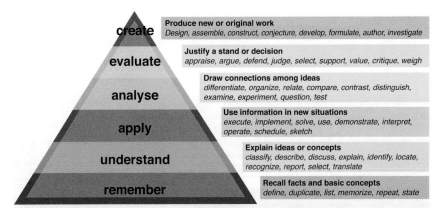

Fig. 6.4 Bloom's educational taxonomy. (Image from: Armstrong, P. (2010). *Bloom's taxonomy*. Vanderbilt University Center for Teaching. Retrieved 27 May 2022, from https://cft.vanderbilt.edu/guides-sub-pages/blooms-taxonomy/. Accessed 28 September 2021; Bloom, B.S. (1956). *Taxonomy of educational objectives, handbook: The cognitive domain.* New York: David McKay.)

higher education, the equivalent to the diploma level you will need to develop your skills of analysis. As this develops you will develop a critical-thinking skills which will become aligned with level 6 studies (degree level).

Most students when writing at level 4 are descriptive. This is mostly about giving information or explaining a theory or stating the order in which things occur. At level 5 you evaluate strengths and weaknesses and weigh one piece of information against another and draw conclusions (Cottrell, 2019).

Levels 6 and 7 depend on more reading and evidence. There will be an expectation that you can search the literature and reference adequately (Pears & Shields, 2019). In addition, you will draw conclusions, synthesise, and evaluate more particularly as you move to level 7/8 where you will generate new ideas.

ACADEMIC INTEGRITY: WHAT IS IT? WHY IS IT IMPORTANT?

Finally, as studying nursing is a professional course it is important that your academic skills develop to ensure that there are no allegations of plagiarism or poor academic practice. Academic integrity is becoming even more important to universities which is based on a moral code or standard of ethics with honesty at the centre. Most students understand what plagiarism is. There are tools that can be used by students and staff which help prevent it and identify it when it happens. Having good referencing and academic skills can help avoid problems. You will need to learn how to give credit where you have used others' ideas as part of your work and learn how to present and interpret other people's ideas within your own work.

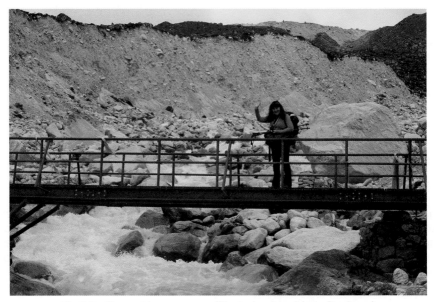

Fig. 6.5   Everest base camp. (Photo by Ann-Marie Dodson.)

Sometimes students form close friendships and do not realise that when working together they could be seen to be 'colluding' if the work is of identical form. There are occasions when working together maybe on a project, is encouraged, but there will be clear guidelines and assessment criteria.

False presentation or contract cheating is very serious, especially if studying nursing as you are expected to be trustworthy and have integrity. This is when you pay someone or a company to do your work. There are many 'essay mills' or businesses too willing to help you. It is totally against any University regulations and your personal data can be misused and sold. There have been cases where the more unscrupulous companies have tried to extort money after the initial payment. Just don't be tempted. You can do this on your own merit and have that sense of achievement as you graduate and become a registered nurse. That day will come, and quicker than you think. Good luck and enjoy. Stop and look back at what you have achieved and what is yet to come. Many doors will open along your journey and take those opportunities if you can (Fig. 6.5).

FUN FACT

Mary Eliza Mahoney was the first African American nurse in 1879. There were 42 students in her class and only four of them finished the nursing programme (her included) (National Women's History Museum, 2017).

References

Armstrong, P. (2010). *Bloom's taxonomy.* Vanderbilt University Center for Teaching. Retrieved 27 May 2022, from https://cft.vanderbilt.edu/guides-sub-pages/blooms-taxonomy/. Accessed 28 September 2021.

Clarke, N. (2017). *The student nurse's guide to successful reflection: Ten essential ingredients.* Maidenhead, UK: Open University.

Cottrell, S. (2019). *The study skills handbook. Macmillan study skills (5th Ed.).* London, UK: Macmillan International Higher Education, Red Globe Publishing.

Equality Act. (2010). *Equality Act 2010: Guidance – GOV.UK.* www.gov.uk. Accessed 29 May 2022.

National Women's History Museum. (2017). *Mary Eliza Mahoney.* https://www.womenshistory.org/education-resources/biographies/mary-mahoney. Accessed 16 May 2022.

Nursing and Midwifery Council (NMC). (2018a). *The code: Professional standards of practice and behaviour for nurses, midwives, and nursing associates.* http://www.nmc.org.uk/globalassets/sitedocuments/nmc-publications/revised-new-nmc-code.pdf. Accessed 29 May 2022.

Nursing and Midwifery Council (NMC). (2018b). *Evidence based practice.* https://www.nmc.org.uk/supporting-information-on-standards-for-student-supervision-and-assessment/practice-assessment/what-do-practice-assessors-do/assessment-of-practice/evidenced-based-assessment/. Accessed 27 May 2022.

Nursing and Midwifery Council (NMC). (2018c). *Realising professionalism: Standards for educations and training [pdf].* London, UK: NMC. education-framework.pdf (nmc.org.uk). Accessed 29 May 2022.

Nursing and Midwifery Council (NMC). (2018d). *The code: Professional standards of practice and behaviour for nurses, midwives, and nursing associates.* http://www.nmc.org.uk/globalassets/sitedocuments/nmc-publications/revised-new-nmc-code.pdf. Accessed 29 May 2022.

Nursing and Midwifery Council (NMC). (2019). How-to-revalidate-booklet.pdf (nmc.org.uk). Accessed 29 May 2022.

Pears, R., & Shields, G. (2019). *Cite them right. The essential referencing guide.* Macmillan Study Guide. Red Globe Press/Macmillan.

CHAPTER 7

Exam Preparation and Revision Tips

Exams, exams, exams! Hands up who loves exams? No? Me neither… I tend to get very anxious; I start having nightmares and I don't sleep the night before. On the day, I have mild heart palpitations, and my hands get sweaty. My mind always went blank during an exam too, until someone told me this amazing tip (see Box 7.1). These are tried and tested tips I used myself to help me through my exams.

Make use of any practice exams your university gives you. Birmingham City University (BCU) always had online practice exams that we could look at to see the layout, etc. of our exam, which I found helped me massively! But if your university does not do this, then have a look for different types of practice exams online just to get your brain flowing. There are some great places, such as Khan Academy, that provide online quizzes and revision sessions for free. Also, the Quizlet app has a lot of revision cards on there too. Find what works for you and go with that. Also, make use of your family and friends! Get them to quiz you and grill you on your exam, it will be awful at the time, but it will stick. All of these little things will make a huge difference to your revision, and you will be shocked at how much you remember the day! However, you need to make sure you're revising the right information too. So, make sure you are using good resources for your revision: anatomy and physiology books, official websites, university resources, libraries etc. Because all this advice is only good if what you're revising the correct information.

Also, make use of your free time to revise. I used to get to my placement an hour early to get an hour of revision in before I started placement! Because every hour counted. It also helped me keep evenings freer to take some time out, and this worked really well for me, but I know it's not for everyone. It's just a small idea that you may not have thought of and is worth trying out.

Objective Structured Clinical Examination

At BCU, we were very fortunate that we only had one objective structured clinical examination (OSCE) in our first year of nursing. (Other fields and universities may differ, and courses may change in structure with time.) I can give you all the tips and advice I can about OSCE and what we did, but your university and wherever you are in the world might do something slightly different, but

---

BOX 7.1 ■ Revision Tips

Tip 1: 'Use all of the lobes of your brain when revising'.
Reading books, articles, journals, etc. Listening to audio books or lectures. Watching videos such as YouTube channels. Talking to others and talking them through your anatomy and physiology. Drawing diagrams/charts and using different colours to write and draw with.
The theory behind this is: During an exam when that one part of your brain goes blank the other lobes are prepared and ready to back it up.

Tip 2: Making simple but important key words and bullet points rather than long-winded sentences that you won't remember. Using flash cards really helps you to remember these short bursts rather than long structured revision notes.
Theory behind this is: Using shorter words will help you remember the important info you need, and you can fill in your own blanks.

Tip 3: Put post-it notes everywhere! I do this. I stick them to the fridge, walls, kettle, wardrobe and toilet. Anywhere I will go and I can see them.
Theory behind this: The random places you leave them, give you a visual reminder to store in your brain.

Tip 4: Revise in shorter sessions. Doing 25 minutes of revision then have a short 5-minute break will be far more beneficial than trying to cram revision in all day long. Make sure you eat well and drink plenty of fluids during too.

Tip 5: Link your revision to objects you will remember. This will make it easier to recall during your exam. For example, I always thought of the alveoli as broccoli branches. Alveoli also sound like Aioli, which reminds me of garlic mayonnaise. These weird ways helped me remember parts of organs better. Find your quirky ways and use them ☺

Tip 6: Eat different snacks whilst revising, chew gum, and have different smells/air fresheners around you to help. The different tastes and smells will link to what you're revising and help you remember on the day of the exam.

---

hopefully, I'm going to give you some good tips to help you cope in your OSCE as well as just doing a run-through.

Our OSCE came in two parts: the first part was a 20-minute anatomy and physiology exam, and I think there were about 10 questions with a mix of multiple-choice questions and one diagram to label. We had four papers out of which we would be given any one, and we didn't know which one we would get on the day, so we had to revise all of them, basically! The choice of paper was either skin, respiratory, cardiology or renal system. I was very fortunate to get skin because I'm not going to lie, it was the easiest exam out of them all (or I thought so anyway). I'm not saying it was the easier exam, but it's just the one that I found the easiest. Someone else might have found respiratory a lot easier, or someone else might have found cardiology or renal a lot easier. But the skin was my thing back then, so I was chuffed when I opened that paper and this gave me confidence following completing this, to do the main OSCE next.

The second part of the OSCE was the actual physical OSCE. For this you had to do a set of observations on a 'patient' – the patient was your examiner, and you had a second examiner in the corner with the little clipboard marking you. I had to go in and pretend I was on placement; pretend I was out there on a ward, and I had to go in and complete:

- A manual blood pressure
- The temperature
- The pulse checks and
- The respiratory rate

Other things they assessed you on were your communication and professionalism during this. And what I would do if these were out of range or abnormal, and luckily, I managed to just set my mind right and think that this is a real-life situation rather than an exam, and I actually was quite calm throughout my OSCE. I don't know how I did this, don't ask me how, but I managed to just put myself in that place, that 'I'm on a ward and this is my real-life patient.' It somehow worked. If you can get yourself into that frame of mind and don't think of it as an exam, that is the biggest tip I can give you. You do this already, you've probably had a placement already, if you haven't had a placement or you've never done all the observations yet, then just practise that routine repeatedly to get used to it. You will be fine. That was pretty much it for our OSCE and that's all we had. I know some people do a speaking exam with this so, you'll have the examiner asking you questions, and you've got to respond and talk through the processes of the body and things like that. The anatomy and physiology stuff, but luckily, we didn't have that. I'm really bad at saying half the terminology with medical processes and medications, haha! I'm not sure how I would have coped if it was a spoken exam actually…

Again, it depends on which field of nursing you're in because they all do something different as well, and I know my friend who was a student mental health nurse; they had a viva (oral) examination. They had to go in and they would quiz you on a load of mental health capacity acts and things like that, it was so very different from what you did as a student. Our exam was pretty straightforward, and I didn't find it too hard at all. However, people were just getting nervous because they knew it was an exam more than anything. Lastly, on a last little note, I'm going to do a very quick brief run-through of how I did my OSCE, exactly step for step and what I did, so that might help you out.

Step one: I walked into the room and said, 'hello my name is Claire and I am a student nurse. Do you mind if I do your observations which include blood pressure, pulse check, temperature, and respiratory rate check?' – professional values are met by introducing yourself and gaining informed consent before starting.

Next step: Ask your 'patient' if they have a preferred name, Mr Smith for example.

And then I'll say, 'thank you that's perfect' and then you've gained your next step, which is getting your patient's preferred name.

Step three: Next you want to do your first bit of observation, so for me, I always did the blood pressure first, I don't know why? But it was just my go-to thing. I explained to the patient what I was doing first, then I got all my equipment, I clean all the equipment down before and after use – infection control is your next step that you have completed.

I would do the manual blood pressure and then I would give the readings, and I would say, 'okay your blood pressure today is 130 over 70 and that is the perfect range because your systolic should be between 100 and 140 and your diastolic should be anywhere between 60 and 90. So, this is in the perfect range'. Step covered, explaining you know the ranges and informing the patient of their observations.

Next step: Inform the 'patient' that you are going to check their pulse. I would go and check the pulse, but you inform the 'patient' that you will be checking the pulse for 2 minutes instead of the standard 1 minute (there is a reason, I swear). Whilst you're checking the pulse (in the first or second minute, it doesn't matter which way around you do this), you will check their respiratory rate as well. So 1 minute was spent checking the pulse, and then an extra 1 minute was spent checking their respiratory rate. The reason you do this is because if you tell someone you are about to count their breathing rate, they will start to adjust their breathing automatically and it wouldn't be an accurate figure you get for this. So, by pretending to check the pulse rate, you can do this unknown to them. However, after you check their pulse rate and respiratory rate, you need to explain what you have done and your findings to them. Again, I told them the ranges of these, so they understood this. So, you would say to them something like, 'Your pulse rate was 78 and that's perfect because it's in the normal range of between 60 and 100. Your respiratory rate was 14 today, so that's great because the range for the respiratory rate is between 12 and 20 per minute'.

Next step: I will do the temperature. I will make sure I clean it all off first. I put a clean cover on it, and I would tell the patient what I am going to do before doing it. Make sure there's no hearing aids or anything else blocking the ear. If hearing aids are worn – ask the patient to remove it so you can do the temperature. Then again, you tell the patient what their results were and the ranges of this.

Final stage: I just end it by saying 'I've now finished all of your observations, they are all in range however, if any one of these were out of range, then I would have to report it back to my mentor and just get them to look into this a bit further, is that all okay and do you need anything else from me?' Because you have to show what you would do if something went wrong. And sometimes on the day, you might get a person with some abnormalities to their observation ranges. So, you would tell the examiner during your OSCE what you have found, and how you would handle it. For example, reporting them to your mentor for further assessment. Done. Cover yourself at all angles.

And lastly, to add to this, we also had to document all our findings on the observation charts; National Early Warning Score (NEWS) chart was used in our OSCE (which may differ and change depending on university guidelines, etc.) We were also marked on writing the NEWS chart accurately, so be vigilant for this ☺

So, my biggest top tips for surviving your OSCE are:

- Practicing, practicing, practicing, practice with your family, colleagues, students, your friends or anyone you can to help you practise this before the exam day.
- Try and think of it like a real-life situation – I know it's almost impossible because it's not a real-life situation and it is an exam room. But try and get into that head space and this will help hugely on the day.
- Know your observations and ranges.
- Make sure the room is quiet if you're doing manual blood pressure so that you can hear it.
- If you struggle with anxiety during exams, try breathing techniques, medication, lavender on pulse points or anything to help keep you calm on the day (within legal limits and not anything you're allergic to, of course).
- I saw a great anxiety tip where you hold a bottle of water and throw it from hand to hand, watching it switch from side to side for a few minutes, this helps you concentrate on something and supposedly helps with anxiety levels. It may or may not work for you.
- Revise the anatomy and physiology using the revision tips in the section as well.

If you're nervous, then you're nervous, don't worry about it because they're going to expect nerves. Also, it's about being safe as well, so if you find a situation where, if you're doing a set of observations like I did and, let's say, you literally cannot get the blood pressure, you're really struggling – that's okay because sometimes you just can't. But as long as you just stop and say to the examiner (be open and honest with the examiners) and just say, 'I'm really sorry, I'm not getting anything here, I can't hear anything,' and then explain what you would do in that situation out on placement to show that you're safe and competent at doing that. That's okay, as long as you say something along the lines, I'm really sorry I can't get this pulse right now, I don't know what's happened I've tried both arms (make sure you try all points you need to before stopping), I can't hear anything, or I can't feel anything. However, if this were me out in placement, I would go and get another nurse or my mentor to come and check it out for me. Then that's it, they just want you to show that you've got things in place for when things aren't quite right, or things are going wrong. To show that you are safe and competent at doing that as well. It's all about best practice and looking after your patient at the end of the day and these things do happen. So, don't worry about it and don't stress about it, don't get so overwhelmed and have a breakdown about it because it's okay.

I know that all these tips helped me, so I'm hoping (fingers crossed) that they help you too. But again, it's about you as an individual and how you learn and remember stuff, that's the best way for you. It might not work for you so it's about finding out about yourself and what works for you.

FUN FACT

There are around 104 nursing professions to choose from (Nurses Zone, n.d.).

Reference

Nurses Zone, (n.d.). *111 Nursing facts.* Retrieved from https://www.nurseszone.in/nurseszone/111-nursing-facts/118.html. Accessed 16 May 2022.

CHAPTER 8

All You Need to Know about Placements: First Year to Management with a Bonus Page of A to E Assessments and Tips for Areas of Placements

The Nursing and Midwifery Council (NMC) pre-registration standards for student nurses (2010) states that students must complete 2300 clinical hours (this may change in future).

> *Practice placements are an essential part of nurse training and will equip you with the skills needed for a successful nursing career. In line with standard 2 of the RCN Nursing Workforce Standards, all nursing students must be supernumerary when in training.*
> ROYAL COLLEGE OF NURSING (RCN, 2021)

At the university, your placement team will arrange your placements. They will consider your location and try to place you closer to home – however, it can be anywhere up to 2 hours away from your home and this will be different across different specialities of healthcare. So, if you are trying to decide which university to choose – think about where your placements might be and how you will get there – this should help you decide.

My placements were mainly around 1.5 hours away on buses from my home. It was very hard to commute whilst on long shifts at the hospital – but it was doable, and I managed it. If you have any concerns about placement, talk to your university placement team, tutor, or mentor. If you have further concerns that are not getting answered by either of these people, you can contact your local union for more advice and help. I'm personally with the Royal College of Nursing (RCN) and they have a whole team to help you, but other unions are available.

Placements can be a very exciting but daunting and nerve-wracking experience, even more so if you have never worked in healthcare before. I was quite lucky that I had 10 years of experience before starting; however, this isn't all that lucky! People often think it is better to be experienced and then go into nursing, but I think those students coming in with fresh eyes are at an advantage here.

BOX 8.1 ■ Tips Before You Start with Placement

- Call your placement about 2 weeks in advance. Introduce yourself and get your first week of shifts from your mentor or the ward manager.
- Ask if you can go in for a visit before you start so that you can meet the team. This will really help your nerves and allow you to see the area you're going to before starting.
- Do a route plan of how you're going to get to and from placement. Check the bus and train timetables or your map if you're driving. Do a practice run before starting so that you can judge how the journey will be.
- When you call your area up, check what staff facilities they have; staff room, kettle, tea/coffee, microwave, and a fridge etc. So, you can prepare your meals for your shift based on what's available to you.

In working in healthcare for 10 years you can get stuck in your ways a little bit and it can be difficult to get out of your 'normal' role. I constantly have to remind myself to stop and take a moment to remember why I am here and what I need to learn. Whatever your experience, placement is all going to be new and scary to start with. You are that newbie! You are having to fit into a new team and get used to that area of working. Once you have passed that first day of introductions and finding your way around, you will feel much better about everything. Here are some tips (Box 8.1) to help you before you start your placements and (Box 8.2) for tips whilst on your placement.

Year 1

On your very first placement, your practice supervisor and assessor (mentors) won't expect much from you. You are at the very beginning and don't know what you don't know yet … I see students panicking that more will be expected of them – please do not panic. Let the team know this is your first-year placement and you will be under the direct supervision of one of the teams on each shift.

If you have healthcare experience already and have done things such as personal care before, tell your nurses this. They can adjust the placement to give you opportunities to do skills that you haven't done before. However, if you have not done personal care before, you will be expected to start there. You will spend a lot of time during your first year working alongside the healthcare assistants and you will be under direct supervision, always. As a student nurse, you will be constantly asking questions during your first year. This is normal. In fact, this is normal for the whole of your career!

- The biggest tip I can give you is to remind yourself you will never physically know it all and no one knows it all – not even top consultants know everything and will have to ask questions themselves. So please be kind to yourself throughout your nursing journey.

BOX 8.2 ■ Tips for Whilst on Placement

- Prepare meals in advance. On your days off, make a big batch of pasta or rice dishes (or whatever you fancy) and freeze them or refrigerate them ready for your shifts.
- Take snacks for your short breaks. I tend to take things like cereal, oat bars, protein bars, fruit, vegetables and hummus.
- Take a little tub with your own milk, tea, coffee and sugar (if you have these) just in case your ward runs out or doesn't provide this.
- Always take a water bottle with you! Stay hydrated. You are on your feet all day long, running around. You need to keep yourself healthy so you can take care of your patients.
- Wear comfy shoes. One of the best tips I have, I have Clarkes – unloop and they are amazing! Like walking on air. But please don't pay full price for these, they are £65! You can get them from the Clarkes factory outlet. Have a look at where you are nearest one is. I got mine for half the price. Most student nurses prefer Clarkes, but I have heard a few students who cannot wear them, and they have Sketchers instead. But just choose what is right for you.
- Shoes must be black or navy, covering your whole foot with a leather or wash-able/hard material. This is from a health and safety point of view; you don't want any bed or hoists running over your toes. Also, you will no doubt get some form of bodily fluids on your shoes, urine, faeces, blood, vomit and more! Your shoes need to be wipeable for infection control purposes.
- Carry a little notepad in your pocket and write down all the things you learn.
- Keep a small A–Z notepad to write all your medications in. As a student nurse you will be expected to learn each medication and all the side effects, contraindications, dose, usage and action on the body.
- Always have a secret stash of black pens in your bag. You WILL lose them…
- Always wear a fob watch. You need this to count the respiratory rate and pulse during your observations. My battery died on mine one day and it was the hardest thing to do without! I had to keep trying to find a watch to use or a clock on the wall to try and count on.
- Don't be offended if your mentor doesn't directly supervise you and they send you off with the healthcare assistants. These are the best people to learn from, they are so knowledgeable. Also, mentors are so busy they have to prioritise patients first. But at the same time if you feel you aren't learning, then speak with your mentor. Ask if there's something you would like to do in particular, you are also there to train as a nurse.
- Ask a lot of questions, no question is a stupid question I promise. Constantly ask nurses why they do certain things, what's the theory behind it. So, you can understand the reasons why things are being done in certain ways. Also, mentors like you to ask questions as this shows that you're interested.
- Ask for pathways – You can ask to go with the pain team, tissue viability team, physiotherapy, theatres etc to build your knowledge and understand how to effectively care for patients.

If you aren't enjoying a particular area and it is getting you down, always remember why you wanted to become a nurse. Remind yourself that you are only on that placement for a certain number of weeks, and you don't have to work there when you qualify. Keep smiling and never let anyone dull your shine!

STORY TIME

I want to share a short story from my own personal experience. My very first placement was a surgical placement on a ward – I had never worked on a ward before, so this was all new to me. I came home crying most days for the first 2 weeks of this placement! Not to scare you … but I hated it. It made me question whether I wanted to be a nurse at all and I felt guilty for not enjoying this area. I can't tell you which part I didn't like, but it was most of it, the conveyor belt system a hospital has: one patient in and one out as fast as possible. Too much noise around me with machines, people etc.; it was hard to concentrate at times. The shift work, I really dislike nights … as discussed in the night shift section. I just didn't like any of it; it wasn't for me.

I really did feel awful about it all… until I met one healthcare assistant. A lovely man who gave me faith again – I saw how amazing he was with patients, and he explained every detail as he went along. I will never forget that kind and caring nature – in fact, I saw him later during another placement in my second year! It was lovely to see his face again. He kept me going to be honest; that, and reminding myself this placement wouldn't last forever. Despite the dislike for the wards, I always gave 100% in everything I did and not one person knew I disliked it. I was always upbeat and positive and threw myself into it all. Every single placement will give you opportunities, if you embrace it enough, which leads me to my first set of tips:

1. Make the most of every opportunity; ask for pathways to different areas and with different teams (e.g. on surgical wards I visited theatres for the day and on my community placement I went to sit with the package of care teams for the morning).
2. Ask questions – and lots of them! No question is ever a stupid one.
3. Write everything down! Have a small note pad and pen in your pocket. I did this, and it saved me from going back and asking my mentor the same questions.
4. Sit with your mentors and get them to sit with you and go through how to document the in-patient notes. My mentor always said: you write from head to toe, from so psychological well-being to pain to sickness to physical skin checks, urine, bowels, feet etc.
5. If you feel confident and trained to do something – get stuck in. However, if you don't, please do not do it and ask for training first – stay safe. ☺
6. Take your time; observe everything you can. You're only a student once, so make the most of this supernumerary status.
7. Ask to go with different members of the multi-disciplinary team (MDT) from healthcare assistants all the way up to management – you will be surprised at what you learn from each member.
8. Don't forget to take your breaks! You are not counted in the numbers (or shouldn't be) and you do not get paid for placements. Take your breaks and look after yourself – be kind to yourself. ♥

Year 2 Expectations

For those of you either just starting nursing or in your first year, this one could be for you. Before starting my second year, I had heard a lot of negativities about it. Students said things like, 'Second year was the worst year of my life', which initially made me a little bit nervous. So, if this is you right now, please don't listen to those comments and just the take second year as it comes. Firstly, I need to add, I have no children. I have no commitments outside of nursing, so the workload wasn't too bad for me. Everyone is different – remember this when reading any tips and advice anywhere.

The one thing I will say here is, second year is a step up and the workload you will get is going up with it. It is a full-on year and if you're the sort of person who leaves things until the last minute, you might struggle.

Small solution – organise and prioritise that workload.

To be honest, all in all, I absolutely loved second year! The modules were so much more interesting and right up my street. I fully embraced it all; even with the challenges I had to face, second year had been my favourite year of it all.

What modules did I have during second year? (Your university will be different, and modules change constantly, so they may not be like this anymore.)

- Nursing Practice 2 exam – Based around three case studies of: cancer, acute abdomen blockage, and multiple sclerosis.
- Nursing Practice 3 exam – Based around three case studies of: diabetic ketoacidosis (DKA), sepsis, and ectopic pregnancy.
- Professional Values and Evidence-Based Practice – Poster presentation and 2000-word assignment based on a patient with dementia.
- Nursing in Society – designing a leaflet on a mother and baby issue with a 1000-word rationale for it and a care plan with a 1500-word rationale for this.
- Maths exam – Drug calculations (it wasn't bad at all!).

We had the majority of these all launched one after the other, and the deadlines, one after the other. You may be faced with the same challenge, but the key is to start the workload as they launch it to keep on top of it. Break down the word load to help you manage it all.

Top tips for second year:

Tip 1: Stay organised – start the work as it is launched to you and break each section down bit by bit.

Tip 2: Prioritise the workload – which ever deadline is due first, do that first.

Tip 3: Check out websites, books, and other useful resources on how to critically analyse academic work. You can always ask your library for advice, as they usually have people to help with academic writing. And a mistake I made was data base searching. ALL wrong, so please seek help from your library personnel. They are amazing and will show you little tips to help you do your research properly and avoid all the mistakes most people make when searching.

Tip 4: Get help – If you are struggling, always get support; do not suffer in silence. There is all the help in the world for you, but you can't receive it if no one knows you're struggling. Speak to someone at the university, your family, friends – Anything other than suffering in silence.

How about those second-year blues?

I definitely felt this for a couple of weeks towards the end of second year. There was a mixture of things all happening at once to make me feel the blues.

Firstly, my grades dropped a little from first year! With the level rising from 4 to 5, I had to raise my standards to match the criteria, and I didn't … I had missed extra points on the smallest of things and that really got to me. Secondly, I was coming to realise I only had a year left after this one. It was making me feel sad thinking about leaving university behind. Spoiler alert – I still grieve for my university life. Maybe I will return one day as a lecturer? Who knows?

And lastly, I had a bit of personal problems with a relationship break up and I had to move right in the middle of my placement. My mother also passed away. I ended up taking a couple of weeks off to get my head together and then get back to it. So, I had a lot of things all at once that were really getting to me. But after a good talking (to myself) and putting myself straight again, I was great! I reminded myself how long it's taken me to get here now, how far I have come, and what I have achieved. I wasn't going to let any of these little things get me down!

Always remember, if you're feeling the blues right now or in the future, remember you're amazing. Look back at your journey and how far you have come! Don't let anything or anyone stop you. You got this!

During this year, you will still be under the supervision of the healthcare professional: your practice assessor/practice supervisor/mentor but this will be a bit more from a distance. They will give you some autonomy and this is your time to put into action all the things you have learnt from your first-year training.

It doesn't matter which area you work in: the human body, anatomy, and physiology are the same. You are going to be using all the clinical skills and your own judgement in every single placement you go to. The only difference is different areas have different ways of running, different technologies, and different people. It's getting your head around the new area, different medications, different treatments patients may have, and different use of equipment – and that's ok.

Remember, no one is out to get you, and your mentors and colleagues all want to see you pass! Just remember to always follow the NMC Code of Conduct and you can't go wrong (unless you're doing something dangerous that risks patient safety of course…please avoid that).

As a second-year student, you will still be expected to ask questions and seek support if you need it. However, you will slowly become more autonomous. You will slowly start saying to your mentor things like, 'I noticed patient A needs this… so I am just going to help with that' instead of 'What should I be doing now?' Once you know the routine of the placement you are working on, you will feel much more comfortable doing this. At the end of the day, you are still a student nurse and still learning; your colleagues shouldn't be expecting miracles from you.

Whilst we are in second year, I think it's a great time to add in 'second-year blues' – a sentence we all dreaded/dread. Second-year blues is a real thing out there and if you do a search on the internet, you will find a lot of students that go through this – BUT please do not panic! If you are already dreading second year from other people's experiences, this is already going to put you on a down-hill spiral. My second year of nursing was *by far* my greatest and best year out of all of them (including being qualified!). I fully embraced university life, got stuck into extra-curricular activities, and really made the most of everything life had to offer me. And this is a great tip for you, too – get stuck in. Get involved in societies and other activities at your university. This is going to keep you so motivated through the years; it did for me. However, I know a lot of people have children and busy home lives and might not be able to do this. So, here are my top tips (Box 8.3) for avoiding those second-year blues and making the most of it all.

Second year is that middle ground. You're no longer a first-year but you're not at the end of the degree either, and I think this is why people struggle. Not only that, but the workload goes up and the marking criteria goes up. So, it's a mixed bag of emotions and no one really tells you how to handle it all. But if you stay focused, and organise and prioritise your workload, you will be fine! And, just to add to your grades, if they do go down in second year, follow my advice on the assignment writing sections and I believe you will improve. The only time you may get asked about grades is if you want to go on and do another course such as a masters or PHD. However, grades don't define the nurse you are. No one asks for your grades when you qualify; at the end of the day, they just want to see that you're a competent nurse. Not one person has asked for my grades yet, so don't get so hooked on grades only. If you're passing the course and being the amazing nurse you are, that's what matters. A grade doesn't consider the sweat and tears you have gone through to revise or sit and write the assignment; it doesn't take into account your home life, stresses, or work life you have going on to get you by, so please be kind to yourself. This grade does not define who you are; the nurse you are will define that. Keep being that caring and amazing nurse!

BOX. 8.3 ■ Tips for Avoiding Second-Year Blues

1. Get your family involved – some of my friends used to teach their children what they had learnt in anatomy and physiology. Make it part of your family routine ☺
2. Whatever makes you happy – do more of that. So, for me, I did meditation quite a lot and breathing techniques when things got overwhelming, and this really helped me. Find what works for you
3. Stay organised – organise what needs to be handed in first and prioritise that workload into management chunks.
4. Little by little – do things in small steps rather than bit lots. I used to do bits of assignments here and there and eventually it was done without even realising it.
5. Use your university support teams to help you – don't be too proud to ask for help.
6. Make sure you are taking time out for yourself
7. Make sure you are eating and drinking (non-alcoholic) well – staying nourished and hydrated will make a huge difference
8. Switch off all technology for a while and just relax
9. It's ok to avoid social media – sometimes it can be so negative. Other times there is so much positivity which can help too. I have a Pinterest account where I keep a load of positive quotes to keep me going.
10. Keep a motivational board at home. Put all your favourite photos, positive quotes and goals on there. Look at it every morning to start your day right
11. Remind yourself why you came into nursing, remind yourself how far you have come so far and all you have achieved! You are doing AMAZING – You got this!

Year 3 Expectations and Entering the Register

The NMC (2019) set out standards for nurses: 'The standards for competence apply to all fields of nursing and are set out in four main areas of professional nursing practice'. These are displayed in Box 8.4.

Congratulations!!! You made it to your third and final year!! You should take a moment to embrace this because there will be students who don't make it this far. But here you are, almost at the end of your student nurse journey. Third-year expectations are the ones you probably want to know most; I know it was for me. Everyone always seems to want to do well on their management placements, but from what I've witnessed, it causes the most anxiety.

First, sit, drop those shoulders, take a big, long deep breath in and out again. You have come this far and there is no reason why you will suddenly start to fail now. Keep doing what you have been doing in second year, but, this time, you will be more autonomous. Your supervisor and assessor/mentors will all want to see you taking more of the lead with patients. They may give you your own bay

> **BOX 8.4 ■ Standards of Competence in Professional Nursing Practice**
>
> - *Professional values*
> - *Communication and interpersonal skills*
> - *Nursing practice and decision making; and*
> - *Leadership, management and team working.*
>
> Within these four areas there are two main aspects to the standards. All nurses must demonstrate their knowledge and competence in both in order to register as a nurse. **These aspects are:**
>
> - The competencies that all nurses across all fields must know and demonstrate; and
> - The specific competencies of each field that an individual nurse is registered in.
> - The combination of both aspects across all four areas is in place to ensure that patients and the public can be confident that all registered nurses will:
> - Deliver high quality essential care to all persons in their care
> - Deliver complex care to service users in their field of practice
> - Act to protect the public, and be responsible and accountable for safe, person-centred, evidence-based nursing practice
> - Act with professionalism and integrity, and work within agreed professional, ethical and legal frameworks, and processes to maintain and improve standards
> - Practise in a compassionate, respectful way, maintaining dignity and wellbeing and communicating effectively
> - Act on their understanding of how people's lifestyles, environments and where care is delivered influence their health and wellbeing
> - Seek out every opportunity to promote health and prevent illness
> - Work in partnership with other health and social care professionals and agencies, service users, carers and families ensuring that decisions about care are shared; and
> - Use leadership skills to supervise and manage others and contribute to planning, designing, delivering and improving future services (NMC, 2019)

to look after, your own case load, your own few patients to see how you do. They will take a step back and allow you to work independently but they will also be there in the background if you need them. I remember my first ever placement of third year and not knowing what to expect. I had the most incredible mentor! In fact, I have been very fortunate with all my mentors; they have all been great and taught me so much. But this mentor wanted to prepare me for my management placement, so I went with the lead nurse, I sat in MDT meetings, and then she said one day, 'Right, Claire, you're in charge today, here you go – off you go…' At the time, I cursed her a little under my breath, but it was the best thing she could have done! This is how I learn and excel! When I am just dropped in at the last minute, I find I swim rather than sink. It's important to know yourself and how you learn best – talk to your mentor about this and work together to get the maximum benefit from your placements.

The way I did my management placement was, first, I watched what my mentor was doing for a good week. I asked questions when I was doing anything I didn't know. My management placement was somewhere I had never experienced before so I had to get used to a new routine and way of working. Once I got the hang of the routine and the way things were done, I started planning the days. I was in the community with the district nurses, so I would get there early to go through the list of patients for the day and organise what we needed for each one, so that when my mentor arrived, it was organised and ready for her to see. This is a really good way to do it if you feel comfortable to do so. If you are on a ward, you can go through the patients you will have and prioritise your day that way. You want to show good leadership and autonomy to your mentor, and this is one way to do this. They want to see you as the nurse, a confident and competent nurse, so they can say, 'Yes, this person can enter the register safely and practice': – if you're showing this, you should have no issues. Management placement is your time to shine and put all of your (almost) 3 years (or 4 years, depending on which route you're taking) into practice. All the knowledge you have gained and all of those clinical skills will now come together. However, it is absolutely OK to feel like you still know nothing! We all feel this at the end: it all starts to get very real and the sudden realisation that, 'in a few weeks' time I will be a nurse,' can be a scary feeling. But this is also the perfect time to talk about any worries you have, anything you don't feel confident in – work on that. Create for yourself Specific, Measurable Attainable Relevant, Time-bound (SMART) goals to work on. Top tips for management:

1. Before starting placement, create your SMART goals. What are your weaknesses? What do you need more training on? Write them out and show them to your mentor when you meet with them.
2. Think about the area you are going to. What can you learn? Is there anything you haven't done that you would like to? Write them down and show your mentor.
3. Take your time, and go at your pace; you are still a student and supernumerary.
4. To be more prepared, research the area before you go in order to get an idea of what they are.
5. Be more autonomous – think for yourself, come up with solutions for the day. Instead of asking what you are doing, go to your mentor and say, 'This is what has happened, and this is what I plan to do about it.'
6. Remind yourself it's okay not to know it all. Nursing is HUGE! You can't know it all. ☺

Placement Specific Tips

These are tips that I picked up on my own placements which may help you before you start yours. Disclaimer: Your placements and experiences may be different to mine. So please research each area separately.

ABDOMINAL SURGICAL WARD

This was my first ever placement and I learnt so much from this area.

Things you might do on this ward are (in no particular order and not limited to): Personal care, including assisting with washing and dressing (including intimate areas), giving medications, assisting with mealtimes including assisting with helping someone eat if they can't do this themselves, changing bedding, observations; blood pressure, pulse rates, respiratory rates, temperature, and capillary refill time. Wound dressings, catheter removals and insertions (if trained to do so), cannula removals/insertions (if trained), IVs (if trained), taking blood (if trained to do so), risk assessments such as malnutrition scores, observation charts (NEWS 2), Skin, Surface, Keep Moving, Incontinence, Nutrition, and Hydration (SSKIN) charts, fluid balance charts, food diaries, manual handling, and pressure relief. You will also complete the patient documents, admission paperwork, and discharge paperwork.

My top tips to help you before you start this placement are:

1. Learn the different abdominal regions.
2. Look up types of abdominal surgery such as ileostomy and colostomy.
3. Learn why people have this type of surgery.
4. Learn different medications for this type of surgery, for example, pain relief and bowel medications.
5. Ask to go to theatres and follow the patient pathway from surgery to recovery and back onto the ward.

STROKE WARD

There are over 100,000 strokes each year in the UK and patients who have had a stroke are at risk of having another one within 30 days of having their first one (Stroke Association, 2021).

On this ward you will do some of the above. But think about communication skills, different communication aids for those who can't communicate as they normally would have before their stroke. Think about what sort of mobility aids and hoists you may use there. Are you trained to use them? An extra risk assessment you will use more regularly in this type of ward is the Glasgow Coma Scale (GCS). This scale is a method for assessing a patient's level of consciousness impairment. It is done by creating a stimuli response (or lack of) to assess this. Some of this includes:

- **Eye opening:** Is it spontaneous? Is it purely to sound, pressure, or none?
- **Verbal response:** Are they orientated, confused, can they use words, sounds or anything?
- **Motor response:** Can they obey commands? Is their flexion (bending a limb) normal – can they bend their arms/legs normally?

(GCS, 2021).

Please, ensure you are trained to do this before you do this alone.

Tips for placement in this type of area:

1. Learn the different lobes of the brain and what they are responsible for.
2. Learn the different types of strokes.
3. Look at different manual handling aids.
4. Look at different aids to help communication in those who have had a stroke.
5. Look at the role of the Speech and Language Therapy team (SALT).
6. Look at different types of food textures; pureed/thickness.
7. Learn different medications for stroke, such as anticoagulants.
8. Learn the signs and symptoms of a stroke and how to treat them.
9. Ask for a day in theatres to see surgery.
10. Ask to go with the SALT team and occupational therapist for the day.

GENERAL PRACTICE PLACEMENT

By far, my favourite of all placements! (P.S.: You can go straight into general practice [GP] nursing as a newly qualified nurse, too; don't listen to the myths that you can't or that you need ward experience first – this is not true.) I went straight into GP as a newly qualified nurse and so can you (if that's where you want to be.) Like with any area, if you want to work there, go for it! Don't listen to other people telling you to experience a different area first; the best thing you can do is just get stuck into what you really want to do. Sorry, I digress . . .

Hopefully, your mentor will give you your own set of patients to see (if you are trained to do the things they are coming in for). I had my own clinics with wound dressings, blood pressure checks, and suture removals. All the things I could do competently and confidently and with my mentor next door – so she was always around for me to go to if I needed assistance. I was still under that supervision but from a distance.

Things you will see during your GP placements: Long-term conditions such as asthma, COPD, diabetes, hypertension. Wound management, clip and suture removals, ECGs, blood taking, cervical screening, a variety of injections including hormone implant injections (Zoladex), sexual health and contraception, height/weight and blood pressures; you may also see some acute chest pain and asthma attacks in clinic, and you may assist in calling an ambulance or providing care to these patients.

Tips for your GP nursing placement:

1. Look up the NICE guidelines for hypertension, diabetes and asthma.
2. Look at different types of wound dressings, clip removals, and stitch removals. The British National Formulary (BNF) has a great wound section table.
3. Look at guidelines for an asthma attack in the community.

TRAUMA AND ORTHOPAEDIC SURGICAL WARD PLACEMENT

This one was one of my favourite ward placements. If I was going to work on a ward, this is where I would be! I found I learnt so much from this placement and gained really great clinical assessment skills here. You will do all the roles as the previous surgical ward placement.

Some of the things you will learn on this placement: pre- and post-operative assessment, a variety of risk assessments, manual handling equipment, different medications and injections, deep vein thrombosis risk, anti-coagulants and types of orthopaedic surgery.

After any surgical procedure you will be doing observations from when they had their surgery to when they recover from it.

Observation timings/the rule of 4 (they may change, as guidelines change):

- Every 15 minutes from time of surgery for 1 hour (4 × 15 minutes).
- Then every 30 minutes for 2 hours (4 × 30 minutes).
- And then every hour for 4 hours (4 × 1 hour).

For example, a patient comes out of surgery at 12.00 p.m. You will do the observations at 12:15 p.m., 12:30 p.m., 12:45 p.m. and 13:00 p.m. Then go onto 30-minute intervals: 13:00 p.m., 13:30 p.m., 14:00 p.m., 14:30 p.m. Then to hourly: 14:30 p.m., 15:30 p.m., 16:30 p.m., 17:30 p.m. After this, if all their observations are stable, they can go to twice daily, morning, and evening observations. This is what I did on the surgical wards I worked in, and may differ from trusts and, with new evidence emerging, procedures may change. The *Journal of Clinical Oncology* (Filson et al., 2018) also shows the best and safest practice is to do more frequent observations.

Observations should include:

- Heart rate
- Blood pressure
- Respiratory rate
- Oxygen saturations
- Level of consciousness using alert, consciousness, voice, pain and unresponsive (ACVPU)
- Temperature
- Pain score
- Urine output

These should also be compared each time to monitor for any signs of deterioration (Sherwood Forest Hospitals, 2019).

Tips for this placement:

1. Learn the bones of the human body.
2. Look at different orthopaedic operations.
3. Ask to see an operation and follow the patient from start to recovery.
4. Look at different medications for orthopaedic: pain relief and the WHO pain relief ladder.
5. Look at different mobility aids and hoists for this area.
6. Ask to go with the occupational therapist/physiotherapist.
7. Look at post-surgery wound care.

Disclaimer: Every trust, every area you go to will have completely different sets of abbreviations. Use these below with caution! It's better to learn the specific

TABLE 8.1 ■ Medical Abbreviations

ABG – Arterial blood gas	IM – Intramuscular
ABX – Antibiotics	IV – Intravenous
ANTT – Aseptic non-touch technique	INC – Incontinent
AVPU – Alert/voice/pain/unresponsive	MDT – Multidisciplinary team
BD – Twice daily	MFFD – Medically fit for discharge
BLS – Basic life support	MUA – Manipulation under anaesthetic
bo/BNO – Bowels open/bowels not open	NWB – Non-weight bearing
CBD – Catheter bag draining	NBM – Nil by mouth
COPD – Chronic obstructive pulmonary disease	NOF/#NOF – Neck of femur/fractured neck of femur
CPR – Cardiopulmonary resuscitation	NORSE – Images linked to Queen Elizabeth Hospital Birmingham
CRP – C-reactive protein	
CSU – Catheter specimen of urine	NAD – No abnormalities detected
CXR – Chest X-ray	OD – Once a day
DHS – Dynamic hip screw	OPA – Outpatient appointment
DM – Diabetes mellitus	ORIF – Open reduction internal fixation
DNAR – Do not attempt resuscitation	POC – Package of care
DVT – Deep vein thrombosis	PRN – As required
ECG – Electrocardiogram	QDS – Four times a day
FBC – Full blood count	R/V – Review
FWB – Full weight bearing	ROC – Removal of clips
GCS – Glasgow Coma Scale	SVU – Self-voiding of urine
GF – Gutter frame	S/C – Self-caring
GI – Gastrointestinal	TDS – Three times a day
HCA – Healthcare assistant	THR – Total hip replacement
HDU – High Dependency Unit	TKR – Total knee replacement
HR – Heart rate	TOC – Transfer of care
HTN – Hypertension	TTO – Tablets to take out
HH – Hand hold	ZF – Zimmer frame

abbreviations to the area you're working in. During one of my placements, they gave me a list of their common abbreviations, which was great! Especially for handover and trying to work out what all the random letters thrown together were. But what I am going to do is add some of the most common abbreviations you'll hear. See Table 8.1.

COMMUNITY REHABILITATION WARD

I really enjoyed this one, too, actually, The staff were great here and it felt very much like I was back working in the nursing home. The ward I was on had a dining room and lounge for patients to sit in, and regular activities going on – it was great! The things you might do on this ward are like the other wards with the personal care, mealtimes, medications etc., but also think about social care with this one. Social workers get very involved in this type of ward as a lot of patients need extra support and care due to living alone and having no family around to help them.

On this ward I saw mainly elderly patients and those who had dementia. One thing I learned during my student days was: 'Aggression isn't a sign of dementia; if someone is showing signs of aggression, upset, restlessness, it's because they want or need something, or it could be a sign they are in pain.' It can be really hard to work out what is causing these issues as the patient may not be able to communicate their concerns, so it's important to try to work out what is causing this distress; show them where the toilet is, give them pain relief, offer food/drinks etc.

Some of the things you may learn on this placement: a variety of medications and injections, a variety of manual handling equipment, dementia care, care planning, communication techniques, risk assessments, rehabilitation of patients back into their homes, risk assessments.

Tips for this placement:

1. Think about communication aids for dementia.
2. Look at the 'This is me' document from the Alzheimer's society.
3. Look at how to create a care plan with a patient/family of the patient.
4. Ask to go with the social workers and occupational therapists.
5. Learn types of medications in dementia.

DISTRICT NURSING/COMMUNITY PLACEMENT

One of my absolute favourites! This placement made me question where I wanted to go when I was qualified. I was very torn between this area and GP. I loved everything about this placement; it was amazing! I had a great team around me, a fantastic mentor, and such lovely patients. I didn't have my own car, so I went alongside my mentor for this placement. I learnt so much from different types of wounds and dressings (I had no idea how many there were!), to diabetes, to catheter blockages, falls assessments to safeguarding. It was amazing.

Some of the things you may learn on this placement: wound management, compression therapy, fall risks, different types of risk assessments, catheter insertion and removals, diabetes/insulin technique, a variety of injections, pressure relief and pressure ulcers, end of life care/palliative care, syringe drivers and medications for this. Working with social workers, occupational therapists, families of patients, hospitals, GPs and podiatrists/chiropodist.

Tips for this placement:

1. Learn the diabetic guidelines.
2. Look at different wound dressings.
3. Look at prevention of falls.
4. Look up pressure relief/ulcer guidelines.
5. Think about lone working and what you would do in an emergency.

HANDOVERS

Now, for me, I have never had a problem with a handover. I don't know why, but I have always just done it and it feels simple to me, but so many people get scared with this. I don't know why, think about why you fear handover so much. The way I think of it is you're just discussing your patients; that's it. So, first things first, of course we cannot do a handover without SBAR.

SBAR stands for Situation, Background, Assessment and Recommendation. When we break it down it means:

Situation: Identify the patient and describe the concerns.

Background: The reason for the patient's admission and their significant medical history and any treatment plans/diagnosis.

Assessment: Observations/vital signs. Clinical impressions/any concerns.

Recommendation: What do you need from the other people you're handing over to? Anything that needs to be done with the patient until the next hand over? (NHS, 2010)

SBAR Example: Patient X in surgical ward. Patient preferred name is patient X and pronouns she/her. Admitted today following surgery for a total hip replacement. No allergies and patient doing well so far. She is on hourly observations and pain relief prescribed which was last given 1 hour ago. Observations are stable so far and up to date and no concerns. They will next need their observations done in 20 minutes and a general well-being check to ensure they are free from pain and pressure relief is given.

Keep it simple and acquire only relevant information. SBAR helps you to structure this.

First tip for handover: for the ones receiving the handover, be on time for your shift. Nobody wants to be waiting around to leave their shift. No one wants to wait for you to come and start work, whether you are on days, whether you're nights, whichever. People just want to get home and people just want to start their shift, so, it's important I think to have an on-time handover and just relieve everybody of their duties and start the shift well.

Second tip has to be communication. You can't have a handover without clear and concise communication. I know it's quite hard to fit in a lot of information in a short space of time so it's important that whatever patients you've got you want to get straight to the point. Put bullet points at the side of your sheet (if you've got a handover sheet) and you want to make notes before the handover on this. So, just put some bullet points of your patients and the important information they need to know. They don't need to know little things like what they wore that day or little things like that. It's more important about the care they're going to receive and anything you need to hand over that are the important bits people need to know. In addition, if those staff members were on the night before or the day before and they know the patients well, it's even more important that you keep it narrow to what they really need to know but also not missing important information.

My next tip is for when you're on shift – make sure you're documenting as you go. If there are really important things that pop up about each patient, make sure you're writing them on your sheet, or make sure you're putting them in your notebook so you remember to hand that over during the handover. It can be quite easy that I've gone into a shift and first thing in the morning something's happened and by the time I'm finishing at eight o'clock at night so much has happened that I can't even remember what I did in the morning. So, it's important that you document everything and that you're writing notes as you go about your patients so that you can give that important handover to the next person.

This tip is all about body language. When you're giving your hand over, don't be the person who slouches in a shy manner, covers their mouth, and talks quietly so people can't hear you. Don't cover your mouth, don't cover your face; you want to stand or sit tall, expand your lungs, and you want your voice to project. I know it is hard and easier said than done. I am that person who is an introvert, so I know it can be difficult, but just make sure your voice is clear. Don't put anything in the way of your face, just open and expand your voice a little bit louder than you would speak if you're a quiet person. If you're quite a loud person maybe tone it down a little bit. It's all about posture as well so make sure you're open and it will just come across a lot clearer.

Lastly, practice and practice. I know it can be quite hard, especially for your very first handover. You're going to be nervous and a bit like 'oh gosh I've got handover; I really don't want to,' and you've been avoiding this forever. But it's really important that you practice, even if you want to practice at home. Get your family members involved. Do a zoom meeting because everything's online now zoom meetings with your uni friends or colleagues or anyone like that. Just have a practice handover where you can all practice with each other. Or if you're doing it in front of your friends and family at home, do the handover to them. Just keep practising it and you'll get into a routine of feeling confident standing and speaking in front of people. However, if you do get anxious and nervous to the point where it's really affecting you, do some things like meditation or breathing techniques, and naming things (tips that are given through this book with anxiety). These techniques will really help focus your breathing and help you relax. Hopefully, it will help you feel a bit more comfortable in that sort of situation as well. But if you're at the point where you really are struggling and nothing is working, you hate life, and you cannot physically do a handover, then speak to your mentors. Speak to other nurses on the ward about how they cope, the things they do, and see if they can suggest anything to help you grow, build, and be able to give even one handover. would be a massive bonus, I think. They could be a huge asset to you, so, just ask. Mainly, it is down to practice. You can't expect to be this amazing handover person right away. Sometimes, I think people take years of practice to do that. I'm not always very good at handovers and sometimes I forget things, and then I go home and panic and ring the ward or wherever I've been, and be like, 'oh, my gosh, I completely forgot to do this.

Will someone do it quickly or hand it over quickly? I'm so sorry'. I've been mortified because I've actually forgot something and luckily it hasn't been anything major. It's just been a little thing, but it made me feel awful at the time so, yes, I absolutely get that and that's okay but just take your time, keep practising, and you'll be absolutely fantastic!

How to Manage a Bad Placement

I'm going to be talking to you all about placements that you might not particularly get on with, you might not enjoy, or you may even just hate completely. I think it needs to be approached because I know a lot of students do struggle on some placements and they're just not enjoying it and they're really struggling to get the motivation to keep going. I'm not going to mention any names, and I'm not going to mention any particular ward areas or trusts or anything like that. I'm just talking about one particular placement area I've had throughout my three years' journey. There was one that I particularly didn't enjoy, I didn't get on with, and I really struggled with. So, when I started University, I had done a lot of healthcare work before, but it was all in the community and I hadn't done many wards. I'd picked up two extra shifts on two different wards before starting university so I could get a general feel of what the wards like, and I think of gauged from that experience that I wasn't going to be a ward nurse. However, I went to university with an open mind; I was motivated, and all that jazz. I went into a ward placement and I just didn't like it. There was nothing bad about the ward. The ward was lovely, the patients were lovely, the staff were (mostly) lovely and my mentor was a very good nurse. That's the main thing: they were a good and safe nurse. If I wanted to go to them for anything, they were so very knowledgeable and they always stuck up for me if I had problems with certain people or patients getting angry or anything like that. I really appreciated that because I didn't like the way some people spoke to me. I thought it was very abrupt and I thought it was very rude. There was no 'please', there was no 'thanks', and with some people you were very much 'the student', and that's it. There was no 'This is Claire'. It was very much 'The student will do this' or 'The student will do that.' I didn't like it, I couldn't get on with it, and after my first day I went home, sat down, and I cried. However, I thought it had taken me many years to get this far and now I'm questioning if I even want to be a nurse. That was tough; that was really tough. To go through that process in my mind and thinking I've made the wrong choice, I've made the wrong life decision, and I thought, 'You know what, it was just a bad day, and I need to go in tomorrow again. I'm only here for 8 weeks, I need to get my head down and pass this placement, and everything will be okay.'

And that was pretty much how it went throughout the whole of that placement. I just put my head down and did everything I could to hide the fact that I didn't like it there. I was really motivated; I was really like, 'Oh, my god, let me do this and let me do that'. I was really proactive, and I was really happy. It was really positive and towards the end of the placement. One of their health care assistants asked me where I wanted to work afterward, and I replied I wanted to go back into the community rather than the wards. She said to me, 'Oh, really?! I would never have guessed you didn't like wards, because you're so active and I thought you actually loved this place'. I thought thank gosh, I'm so glad that came across like that because that's how I wanted it to be, and I didn't want it to affect anybody around me just because that's my personal preference. I'm going off-track now but one of the lecturers during our first year said a fantastic quote. In class we were talking about being on the wards and how has our placement been. There was a question about patients and the question was about having a difficult patient or having a challenging patient and how to manage that. The lecturer stopped what he was doing and he said, 'Is that patient challenging or is that your perception because you have had a bad day or something has not gone your way?' I thought to myself, wow, he's so right because what one person perceives to be one thing, another person will take that completely differently. Your perception can be altered if you wake up in a bad mood and start your day off wrong. Everything is maybe going to annoy you that day if you're stressed or if you're anxious. But, if you're awake, you're waking up happy, you're refreshed, you've had a good night's sleep, you're eating well, you're drinking well, and you're in a positive mood, you're going to take things on the chin, be more relaxed about things, and carry on. Sometimes it is our perception and how we're feeling. We have to remind ourselves that if we are faced with what we think is a 'challenging patient' or a 'difficult patient' (I really don't like those terms), or if we are faced with a patient that we're not getting on with, we have to sit back, take deep breaths, and remind ourselves, 'This patient has been dragged from their home, come into a hospital, and they haven't got their loved ones around them. We've taken their medication from them, we've taken their 'normal' mealtimes from them, we've given them this routine of you will eat it this time and you will have your medications at this time'. We have to think about this person who is unwell and they're in hospital without anybody, with these new people coming at them and they're going to be scared, they're going to be worried, nervous, anxious, they might want to take the frustration out on you but without realising it. We must remember that they are a patient, and we have to care for them and maintain our NMC code of conduct at all times. So, that if you are facing a 'challenging' or 'difficult' patient who is affecting you emotionally, take a step back and address your thoughts and feelings apart from this patient. Speak to your mentor and have a debrief or speak to your colleagues or meet your placement team. If you need to, reflect on it all and do everything you can to distance yourself from your emotions and nurse that patient effectively. Obviously, if someone's physically abusing you, that's not okay; we don't tolerate abuse as nurses (or we shouldn't). That's not okay, and they need to be told, but if it's just general agitation, then that behaviour from a patient is understandable.

If it's just the ward that you don't like, like me, make the most of every single opportunity. You just need to really get stuck in, ask a lot of questions, and make the most of that placement because every single placement is a completely new learning opportunity whether you enjoy it or not. You're going to get some extra skills and you might learn something. You can take that on board as well because you can think, okay, I don't like that, so in the future when I'm a nurse and I'm qualified I won't do that in my practice. Just please make the most of everything you can. However, if you feel like you're not learning as much on the wards because you feel like you're doing one task, like washing patients all day every day and not performing your other skills, and you're an expert on washing patients now, and that's all you've done for 6 weeks, then you need to tell your mentor 'Listen, I really want some experience in this skill or that skill; would it be possible to put that in place for me?' It's just the way you approach these things with your mentor as well, so you could say to them, 'I could really learn a lot from you, could you show me how to do this as I really want experience in this and I'm only here with you for so many weeks and I really want to get those skills'. Just remember to be polite and I'm sure they'll accommodate it. It's about being open and honest as well, having those open and honest conversations with people around you in a professional, polite manner.

Now the tricky one is if your mentor is the problem. We are all human beings and we all have somebody we're going to clash with. There might be a personality clash, our characters clash and it does happen out there. I've had that before, too, but luckily not so much on placement. I worked somewhere in the world, and I had to work with a doctor in a clinic one day and this doctor didn't treat me very well. They spoke down to me, they didn't say 'please' and they didn't say 'thank you' and I sort of felt like a little bit used and abused by them. There were things this doctor could independently do, but used me to do them. I had other things I had to do and was constantly put down. I'd always go out of my way to do things daily, but it was never enough. If I did everything the right way, this doctor would find something to pick at. This behaviour occurred with everyone. It wasn't just me, and there were quite a few complaints made about this doctor. I'm not 100% sure why it was always being done, and I never confronted this issue with the doctor. That's not me, so I killed this doctor with kindness instead. I want this little example to illustrate to you that sometimes we just don't get on with people, but you still must make the most of that opportunity. However, if you get to the point where you feel like you're being bullied or you feel like you're really struggling and you can't work with this person anymore, please speak to your placement department at university, speak to your placement practice managers on placement, and you could even speak to the sister on the ward if you felt comfortable with doing that. I've known students who have been pulled off that ward because it's been really unsafe for them numerous times, so the universities do have things in place for you and hopefully they will help you. We just have to be mindful that our mentors are really stressed right now, and you know you've seen the impact of the staff shortages out there as well. It is stressful, they are going to be really struggling, they're going to be at loose ends out there, and they're going to be trying to do a million and one things at once. To top off their workload they have to have a student to mentor, so they might snap at you sometimes – they might just get a bit agitated – and so we just have to take into consideration that they're going to have a lot going on and not to take things personally. Hopefully, you can cheer them up, make their day, and help them a little bit. If you feel comfortable talking to your mentor, you could say, 'Listen, I just want an open, honest conversation with you as I feel like you're being just a little bit rude with me; is there anything I can do to help? Or, if there's anything I can improve on or build on, please let me know'. You could also add, 'I want this relationship to be a good one as I'm only here for 8 weeks and I really want to learn from you because you're a really good mentor and you are knowledgeable,' etc. I know it might not seem like much, by saying this, and you might not even want to say it, but it tells that person about (1) their behaviour toward you without going in all guns blazing and (2) your professionalism, which might make them realise what they are doing and change as a result. I think they would probably appreciate that a lot more than you going to the practice placement manager or the person in charge to complain first. Then if you still have problems or if you're not comfortable doing that then speak to your team/managers and sort it all out. It's not fair if you're struggling and it's not fair if you're not getting the best learning experience from your placements because you're only there a short time and you need to learn as much as possible before you qualify. Once you're qualified you might be thrown in at the deep end so just take that on board and hopefully sort it out. All in all, I've had good placement experiences and I can say, despite not being a ward nurse, I've thrown myself into it and I've had good experiences from it. I've learnt quite a lot from every single place I've been.

You are there to learn, gain experience, and train. And the new students who are just starting don't get the bursary anymore, and are paying for this experience. You all want to get what you are paying for, you want to learn and want to train, and you're not going to want to have those poor experiences out there.

STORY TIME

I'm going to tell you a little story because it might help you decide whether to speak up or not. I worked in a care home a fair few years ago and I hadn't been there very long, but I'd worked with one particular healthcare assistant (HCA) and I didn't like the way she spoke to patients, I didn't like the way she was rough handed with patients. I didn't like working with her. I didn't agree with anything she did; she had no compassion, no empathy, she had nothing. She didn't seem to care about the patients but that wasn't enough evidence for the manager to do anything about it. So, I sat back and said nothing just like everybody else did (because everybody else knew exactly how this woman was as well). Then this one day, just by chance, I witnessed this HCA physically grabbing a patient by the arm and dragging them off the chair, forcing them to go the toilet. And that is just a huge no, and the times I *do* speak up are to protect my patients. If I see anyone abuse a patient, colleague, friend, family. I will be there for them. So, after witnessing this, I walked into the manager's office and wrote a full statement of everything I had just witnessed. I wasn't the only person in that room because she did it quite openly in a lounge where there were family members and other care staff beside me. However, because I'd gone to the manager, because I wrote my statement and spoke up about it, everybody else came forward. Everyone else was so scared to say anything because they didn't like her, and they knew what a horrible person she was, and they feared her. They didn't want to speak up because of that but, because I came forward and spoke up, it encouraged everybody else to speak up too. I'm so thankful that I did and I'm so glad that everybody else did. She was removed from the building, and she was struck off, never to touch a patient again. Although it was scary, it was a proud moment because I protected my patients and empowered the staff to be able to speak up as well. So, you have to speak up sometimes; you have to protect your patients. That is what you're there for; you're an advocate for your patients. It's in the NMC code and if you're just turning a blind eye, you may as well be committing the crime as well because you're not following the NMC code of conduct which were supposed to do as nurses and you're not protecting that patient.

I just wanted to share that story because it might hopefully inspire you that if you see abuse happening out there or if you see this culture out there, you need to report it. Even if you wait until after your placement is finished to report it. So that they don't know it's you and you can do it anonymously, so it doesn't affect your placement. Please do it either way because you are the one person who will stop it in its tracks from happening to others.

Let's end on a high. All in all, I've had fantastic placements; like I said, I haven't had any issues really. I hope that you have amazing placements and I just want to reiterate that if you have one bad day, it doesn't mean a bad career. If you have one bad placement, it doesn't mean you have to work there. You've got a whole amazing, fantastic career of being a nurse ahead of you and you're going to find an amazing job. A lifelong career ahead of you, so embrace it all.

Medications Rounds with Your Mentor

This part of your day can be both terrifying and exciting. It's terrifying because if you made a serious mistake it can result in harming a patient! However, it's exciting because it's another clinical skill under your belt to learn as a student nurse and you are going to be so chuffed with yourself when you remember the medication names and what they do.

Every university is different in what they do and how they train, so always check your university guidelines (as always) with everything.

At Birmingham City University during the years of January 2017 – November 2019, we had a certain number of medications to learn for every placement we had. The first year we started off with five medications for each placement; then moving on into the second and third year we had 10 medications for each placement. The things you had to know about each medication were:

- Name and dosing of the drug
- Side effects and contraindications
- How the drug works in the body (mechanism of action)

One thing I did to help me learn different medications was to go through the BNF book and make flash cards for every single category of medication. I'm not going to lie; it took what felt like forever to do! But I used short bullet points and lots of different colours to make them and it really did help me remember the types of categories and what they do in the body; Use the tips for exam revision to help you remember these too. But find the best way for you and how you learn because we all learn differently, after all.

The more you do the medication rounds with the nurse, the more familiar you will become with the medications: Like everything we do, it's time and practice.

Some important points to remember during your medications round:

- You must not give any medications without your practice supervisor around. You must always be supervised when giving *any* medication.
- Ensure you are checking the 5 Rs of medications:
  - Right patient: check their name and DOB against the medications chart and their wrist band.
  - Right medication: Is it the right medication for the condition?
  - Right dose: Is the dose right for what they need?
  - Right route: oral, nasal, topical, rectal etc.
  - Right time: Is it being given at the time it should be?
    (Hanson and Haddad, 2020)
- Does the patient know what they are taking and why they are taking it? Don't forget – informed consent.
- Ensure you can read a prescription! If it's not legible, take it back to the doctor and get them to re-write it! Don't just assume and give the wrong thing.
- Don't leave your medications trolley unlocked when you leave it.
- Don't leave the medications trolley/cupboard keys lying around.
- Ensure medications are given with or without food as prescribed.
- Some medications NEED to be exactly on time, such as Parkinson's medications.
- Ask patients if they are on any non-prescribed medications which may interact with their prescribed medications.

- DOUBLE check any contraindications of medications, such as Warfarin which interacts with grapefruit juice! Make sure the patient knows this and there is a clear sign on their bedside for others to know too.
- If you see something not quite right, speak up or report it if needed. I remember working alongside one mentor who got so distracted they kept putting a few tablets in a pot of medication when it was only supposed to be one! So, I had to keep saying, 'You've already put that one in there!' Overdosing or undertreating a patient can result in harm to your patient – so please be vigilant and do not get distracted yourself.
- Not to scare you here, but … Always remember, just because something is prescribed by a doctor, doesn't mean it's correct … mistakes are made, and things are missed, so always double-check everything because it will be just as much your error if you have given something that was not right!

There are a couple of different types of medication prescribed:

- Patient specific direction (PSD)
  - This is a specific prescription done by the prescriber specifically for that patient and their condition.
- Patient-group direction (PGD)

  This is a different type of 'prescription' which is for a whole group of people having the same thing. This is what we use for vaccine clinics such as flu and COVID-19 vaccines at the minute.

  This is licensed through NICE guidelines and medication authorities and then signed by your prescriber in your area (mine would be a doctor/GP) and signed by yourself to say you are competent and understand all of the requirements to give that medication.

For a PGD, you can access this online to have a look at. Just type into your search engine: 'PGD influenza or COVID-19', and you should find it.

On the PGD it gives specific instructions about who can give the vaccine, inclusion and exclusion criteria of who can have it, side effects, registered body named and signed by and then a back page for staff to sign and then a doctor must sign to say you are safe and competent to give the vaccine/medications.

Areas you will see PGDs the most are places such as GP placements, sexual health placements, and vaccine clinics. You should only give medications if you are trained, competent to do so, and have the correct registration required on the PGD. If you do not have this, you need to give medications under the PSD issued by the doctor instead. So, for our healthcare assistants, for example, they can't give under a PGD, but they will help with our COVID-19 vaccine clinics. Our GP will have to print out a whole list of PSD for every single patient and sign to say the HCA is okay to give these. The HCA will then be under the direction of the doctor for this – I hope that makes sense. But it's basically a piece of A4 paper with a list of patient names on it, what vaccine/medication they are having, and signed by the doctor to say they are safe to have this. Each area will be different in how this is done.

With a PGD, a nurse is signing to say they are competent and trained to give it themselves and should do all the checks for each patient themselves when they arrive.

Medications Adverse Reactions Reporting

Any medications that cause adverse effects should be reported through the yellow card scheme (2021). This is run by the Medicines and Healthcare products Regulatory Agency (MHRA) which is the executive agency of the Department of Health and Social Care. It's an online website that anyone can access from home or work. The agency keeps an eye on all of the reactions so that they can have an early warning about any medications which may need to be investigated. All medicines can be reported, such as:

- Vaccines
- Blood factors
- Immunoglobulins
- Herbal medicines
- Homeopathic remedies
- Medical devices available on the UK market and concerns related to e-cigarette products

The Royal Pharmaceutical Society (n.d.) has produced professional guidance on safe and secure handling of medications with some great advice:

2.1 The guidance in this document takes a quality management systems approach to the safe and secure handling of medicines.

2.2 The basic governance principles described in this document can be applied to all healthcare settings.

2.3 The four core governance principles that underpin the safe and secure handling of medicines are; 1. Establish assurance arrangements. 2. Ensure capability. 3. Seek assurance and 4. Continually improve.

2.4 These governance principles are to be applied to each aspect of the safe and secure handling of medicines.

Also, within this document, it provides guidance on:

- Storage of medicines
- Controlled drugs
- Operating theatres

The NMC also has guidance for nurses and nursing associates on their website; take a look and familiarise yourself with these.

WHAT IS BLOOD PRESSURE?

Here is a little explanation of what the numbers mean and how blood pressure works. So, if we go back to the bare basics and think about the heart, the heart needs to pump at a certain rate, certain depth and a certain pressure to get that blood flowing around the body to make sure that there's enough oxygen and nutrients get into your organs and tissues to keep you alive basically. So blood pressure is literally the force that your heart is pumping that blood around to make sure it's reaching those organs. When you measure blood pressure, blood pressure ranges will go up and down all the time depending on what you're doing; if you're stressed, if you're walking about and if you're running, your blood pressure is going to change according to what you're doing, so don't worry if you're checking your blood pressure and you're getting these varied results. As long as your patients' blood pressure is not going high all the time, especially when they're resting. However, if that's happening then that's when you need to get a further assessment of this done by a nurse/doctor.

So, how is blood pressure measured? You'll always have two numbers in a blood pressure reading. The top number is the systolic number or systolic pressure and then the lower number is the diastolic pressure or the diastolic number. The systolic number is the highest level of pressure coming out of your heart and pumping around your body and then the diastolic is the lowest level of pressure coming through the arteries. What this is doing? If you think about your arteries, you've constantly got this flow of blood going through the arteries every single second/minute. The systolic (high/top) number, (what we're measuring on a blood pressure machine) is the stretch of the artery. So, you've got that first burst of blood going through the artery and it's that stretch, so how much pressure is that stretch in the artery as the blood flows through. If you imagine blowing up a balloon, it's the measurement of that stretch in the balloon as you blow it up more and more.

Next we have the diastolic (lower/bottom) number, which is the recoil of the artery. So, how much pressure is left behind once that blood's gone through. You measure in first stretch and then how much pressure is left behind once it's gone through the artery if that makes sense. Imagine now letting the air out of that balloon you just blew up. That's the recoil of the artery and that's what's being measured - It's what is left behind.

So, if the top number's really high, if you think about you're artery stretching really far (like blowing up a balloon too much and 'pop') it could put you at risk of bursting the artery. Also higher risk of heart attack and a stroke.

It's not good to have that high pressure constantly or if there's a lot of blood left behind. If that number's high, you've got a lot of stagnant blood which means you're going to be more risk of blood clots forming and a build-up in the arteries making you more at risk of heart attacks and strokes again. This is why it's really important to get that pressure as normal as possible. So I hope that's helped you understand blood pressure and why it's so important.

Disclaimer: every trust, every area you go to will have completely different sets of abbreviations. Use these with caution! It's better to learn the specific abbreviations of the area you're working in. During one of my placements, they gave me a list of their common abbreviations, which was great! Especially for handover and trying to work out what all the random letters thrown together were. But what I am going to do is add some of the most common abbreviations you'll hear:

Common generic abbreviations for medication administration – see Table 8.2.

Package of Care When Discharging Your Patients

I really need to add this here because this was a huge learning curve for me, and it made a HUGE difference in how I discharged patients, and I helped the nurses around me with this too. Not a lot of people will get the opportunity to do this, so I really want to share this knowledge with you, and I hope that this will enable you to go out and help others as a result.

STORY TIME

Throughout my time as a healthcare assistant, student nurse and now qualified nurse there is something I have picked up on that I would love to share with you and my ideas around this to protect the future of our patients.

Firstly, working as a care assistant in a residential home for the elderly, we had a patient who was discharged back into our home, and they ended up with a readmission. Now, at this time, I was unskilled, I wasn't sure why this happened, and I didn't think to question it.

My next step was as a student nurse. Throughout my time on the wards during my first and second year, I watched patients being discharged and wondered if it was safe to do so. Not only this but seeing the number of patients that were medically fit to be discharged and had nowhere to go, due to a package of care needing to be put in place and this not being done in time for them which then held up the discharge process. These patients needed extra care and time, but it was taking longer than usual for this to be set up. This time I asked the questions to my mentors, 'Why is this patient waiting so long? What's the process?' and their response was always, 'We are waiting for the package of care to be approved' or 'We have had the referral form bounce back to us as it wasn't filled out properly'. I thought, well, what's gone wrong for this to happen? I wanted to look a bit more into this, and I set up a day to 'shadow' the continuing healthcare team to see how the referral process works and gain a bit more knowledge so that I can take this with me to help others and help patients in the future. It was eye-opening to see how much detail is really needed on the referral form and the process it goes through to accept and find suitable needs for a patient. I had no idea! But then, how would we know if we don't get taught this?

TABLE 8.2 ■ Medical and Medication Abbreviations

b.d. = bis die – twice daily

t.d.s. = ter die sumendus – three times daily

t.i.d. = ter in die – three times daily

q.d.s. = quatro die sumendus – four times daily

q.q.h. = quarta quaque hora – every four hours

o.m. = omne mane – every morning

mane = morning

o.n. = omne nocte – every night

nocte – night

p.r.n. = pro re nata – as required

stat. = immediately

a.c. = ante cibum – before food

p.c. = post cibum = after food

Routes of medications:

p.o. = per os – by mouth

n.g. = nasogastric

s.l. = sublingual

IV = Intravenous

IM = intramuscular

Subcut = subcutaneous

p.r. = per rectum

p.v. = per vagina

gutt. = eye drops

occ. = eye cream

e/c = enteric coated

m/r = modified release

Drug abbreviations:

ACE = Angiotensin-converting enzyme

GTN = Glyceryl trinitrate

MAOIs = Monoamine oxidase inhibitors

NSAID = Non-steroidal anti-inflammatory drug

SSRIs = Selective serotonin reuptake inhibitors

ADHD = Attention deficit hyperactivity disorder

AF = Atrial fibrillation

AIDS = Acquired immunodeficiency disorder

BMI = Body mass index

BP = Blood pressure

CNS = Central nervous system

COPD = Chronic obstructive pulmonary disease

CSM = Committee on safety of medicines

CVA = Cerebrovascular accident

CVD = Cardiovascular disease

ECG = Electrocardiogram

GI = Gastrointestinal

HF = Heart failure

HIV = Immunodeficiency virus

HRT = Hormone replacement therapy

IHD = Ischaemic heart disease

INR = International normalised ration

LVF = Left ventricular failure

MHRA = Medicines and healthcare products regulation agency

MI = Myocardial infarction

NHS = National Health Service

NICE = National Institute for Health and Clinical Excellence

NPF = Nurse prescribers formulary

PGD = Patient group directive

RTI = Reproductive tract infection

UTI = Urinary tract infection

VF = Ventricular fibrillation

VT = Ventricular tachycardia

WHO = World Health Organization

WPW = Wolff-Parkinson-White (syndrome)

This is a regular comment throughout this book and what I realised is university gives you the bare foundations to make you a registered nurse; what you do with that is what makes you the nurse, a good nurse.

What is package of care firstly? Package of care or NHS continuing health-care is what you are entitled to if you have a serious illness or disability. Costs of care are covered by the NHS to you which includes things such as personal care and is referred by a healthcare worker. These are put in place when a patient is being discharged back into the community and needs care. Sometimes if a person was well before going into hospital, but, following admission, they suffer illness/disability because of a health decline such as a debilitating stroke. They may be entitled to this, so this has to be put in place before the person is sent home or they won't be safe to be home alone, and this can result in a readmission.

During my management placement as a student nurse, I worked in the community with the district nurse. This is where I saw how it can *actually* affect a patient and just how wrong an unsafe discharge can go. There was one case in particular, which I won't go into too much detail about due to maintaining confidentiality. This was a patient who was quite unwell; they were classed as end of life, they were completely bed-bound, very weak and couldn't eat and drink alone as they normally would and had a grade 3 pressure sore to their sacrum area. This patient had neither family nor friends to look after them at home.

They already encountered repeated readmissions to hospital as they hadn't received the right level of care required for their discharge, and here they were again. This patient was about to be discharged with only four calls a day and needed a lot more. We called the hospital and spoke with several nurses and the manager. My mentor asked them, 'Do you know what four calls a day is and what this entails?' They did not know at all what this meant. Let me tell you what this package meant that this person had; four calls a day which were 20-minute calls each, where the carer visits them to check they are okay, prepare food and assist with toileting needs. Those were day calls, not night calls. This patient had a grade 3 pressure ulcer, they needed a minimum of four hourly repositioning to prevent this from breaking down even more as per NICE guidelines (2014). This patient could not reposition themselves and needed someone to physically help them. They also needed someone to help with drinking and eating, changing their incontinence pad, washing and dressing, cooking etc. Not only that, this patient was on end-of-life care and needed 24-hour monitoring as they were high risk of falling out of bed. This person having 4 × 20 minutes calls a day was not enough and extremely unsafe and more likely to cause another readmission.

It is evident that this happens frequently, and many healthcare professionals don't really know what a package of care really entails and how it will meet the needs of their patients. It turned out that the person filling in the referral hadn't added that this patient was bed-bound or end-of-life on the form, so they got the wrong package of care for their needs. Attention to detail is key to this.

There seems to be an ongoing missing step between the acute sector and primary care/community which is why I am writing this today. In June 2019 the Care Quality Commissioners released their stats on 'adult inpatient survey', and this found that patient discharges had negatively deteriorated since 2017.

Furthermore, one in five patients stated their family or home situation was not considered during discharge planning. Alongside this, 41% of patients were delayed discharge which can have a negative effect on their health outcomes (CQC, 2019). But why is this important? Not only are patients at risk of readmission, they also have the psychological impacts of going back to hospital and the extra workload of healthcare professionals as a result. In addition, the British Geriatrics Society (2017) published that deconditioning of older people over the age of 65 years can happen within a few hours of them lying on a bed, trolley, or sitting in a chair. Not only this, but patients are at a higher risk of acquiring a hospitalised infection as a result too which can cost a higher mortality rate as well as added NHS costs (NICE, 2016).

But for me, it's not about the statistics and cutting costs, it's about protecting patients and ensuring we are giving them the best care possible and the best quality of life possible. So, I ask of you, please ensure your patients are safe to discharge, ask about their home life and if they have support at home. Furthermore, if they need a package of care put into place, please ensure every single detail, in full, is added to the form. And lastly, find out what that package of care entails and if this really does meet the needs of this patient. Because three calls a day may only be 3 × 20 minutes only and your patient might need more than this. This may take you a little longer to write out, but it will save you and the patient a lot of unnecessary stress and prevent a failed discharge later on. Most of all, it could save a patient's life.

Thank you so much for your time; let's protect patients, one safe step at a time.

Risk Assessments and Charts

This section will cover some of the risk assessments and charts you may come across out on placements. List is not limited to, and these may differ from trust to trust. This is a very brief guide for your information, and you will gain more knowledge of these whilst out on placement.

A to E Assessments: The skills you use will include the A to E assessment: airway, breathing, circulation, disability and exposure.

Airway: An obstruction of the airway is an emergency, and you need to get help As Soon As Possible (ASAP)! We assess the airway from the moment we walk toward a patient. We say hello and they respond to us – this is how we know the airway is clear. If they look pale, lips are blue, and they are struggling to talk in full sentences, or their airway is making a noise when the patient breaths – this could be a sign of obstruction of some sort, or the airway is compromised in some way.

Signs of partial obstruction could be: Gurgling sounds, stridor, wheezing, bubbling, choking, gasping for air, coughing, unable to speak in full sentences. **Signs of FULL obstruction could be:** Being unable to speak, having no chest movements, difficulty in breathing, gasping for air, high-pitched wheeze, cyanosis, stridor and unconsciousness.

Breathing: Look, listen and feel technique. What's the respiratory rate? How much effort is being used? Is there any chest abnormality? Is their breathing making any sounds? Does this patient have any breathing disorders/asthma/COPD etc.? Respiratory signs of distress: cyanosis (blue skin or lips), sweating, use of accessory muscles, rattling/wheezing sounds, unequal rise and fall of the chest.

Normal Respiratory Rate: 12 to 20 respirations per minute (Royal College of Physicians, 2017).

Circulation: Is the patient looking paler than usual? Is their skin cold/clammy? Blood pressure/heart rate/Capillary refill time all, okay? Is this patient clutching at their chest in pain? Remember other conditions can cause an issue with circulation as well.

Signs of circulatory issues: cyanosis, pale and cold skin, have they passed enough urine? Irregular pulse rate, patient consciousness levels altered.

Normal capillary refill time: Under 2 seconds

Normal Heart rate: 51 to 90 beats per minute

Acceptable systolic rate: 111 to 219 mmHg (Royal College of Physicians, 2017). However, you will be taught 'normal' is between 100 and 140 mmHg and to report any changes outside of these ranges.

Disability: Is the patient conscious? Check the patient is alert, conscious, do they only react to your voice, pain, pupil size, are both equal and do they change with light? Is there a medication affecting this patient, for example, is morphine causing respiratory depression? Or overdosing of medications? Is the patient diabetic or are their glucose levels too high/low?

Exposure: To examine the full body of the patient for any abnormalities; skin reaction, rashes, signs of infection, continence, assessment of venous thromboembolism (VTE) and nutrition screening (Resus, 2021).

However, just doing a set of observations won't give you the whole picture. For example, during my time as a student, I had a patient who literally looked like they were about to die. The colour of their skin was very grey looking, they were screaming in agony with pain from somewhere and they started projectile vomiting this yellow/green bile. This person was not okay … yet when I did their observations (once I had cleaned them up) they were all completely normal. But clearly, this patient was severely sick. A few doctors, second opinions and then the critical care team later, this patient was very sick… he had an ischemic bowel and later died that night. ☹

So, no matter what you take from all of this, if your patient is not well, if they look physically sick, if anything is making you think. 'I need to get a doctor' – you get that doctor. If you don't agree with a decision a doctor makes, it's perfectly ok to get a second opinion! Which is what I had to do in this case. Just because a doctor is highly educated, with lots of experience, doesn't mean that they get it right all the time. Not to put any doctors down, because they are all fabulous! But there are occasions where you might see this, like I did. You're the one who looks after that patient every day, usually, way more than all the doctors around you. You will know your patient inside and out, so please voice your concerns if you have them. Your patient should always be your top priority over everything else so think of each patient as your own family member and what you would do for them.

Bed Rails Assessments: This is used to assess whether bed rails are needed for a patient. Bed rails shouldn't be used in those with delirium as they are more at risk of an injury/getting stuck.

Falls Risk Assessment: This is used to predict the likelihood of a person having a fall. Things to look out for are patient medications (are they causing drowsiness?), is the patient blood sugar levels stable, is their blood pressure stable? What type of shoes are they wearing, do they fit well? Does the patient have oedema to legs/feet? Are there any environmental factors that may trip the patient such as wires and rugs?

Malnutrition Universal Screening Tool (MUST): This is a screening tool which can identify adults who may be suffering from malnourishment, or risk of or they may be obese. This tool also has management guidelines. The five simple steps in this guide are:

- **Step 1:** Use weight and height measurements to calculate the BMI score – if unable to get these measurements you can use an alternative (Mid Upper Arm Circumference [MUAC]) which is measuring the distance from the bony protrusion on the shoulder (acromion) and the point of the elbow (olecranon process) and mark the mid-point (midway up the arm). Then measure around the arm at the midpoint, this will give you the measurement:

  MUAC below 23.5 cm = BMI is likely to be under 20

  MUAC over 32 cm = BMI likely to be over 30

- **Step 2:** Document the percentage of any unplanned weight loss and score using the table on MUST tool. Equation: weight loss amount in kg divided by the kg and multiply by 100.

- For example, if someone has lost 5 kg, their normal weight was 60 kg = $5/60 \times 100 = 8.3$

- **Step 3:** Document if patient has been acutely unwell recently and if there may have been a reduced nutritional intake or none recently.

- **Step 4:** You add all the scores together from the MUST chart to show their overall risk of any malnutrition

- **Step 5:** Depending on what the risk score is, will show you what to do next, such as food diary, documenting, how to improve nutrition, and referrals to dieticians if needed (BAPEN, n.d.).

Moving and Handling Assessments: This is designed to assess patient safety but also for staff safety when they provide any care to a patient. It will assess what level of care a patient needs and type of equipment needed such as slide sheets and hoists.

NEWS 2 Charts: This is to assess patient deterioration. You document the observations we discussed at the start with A to E assessments, onto this chart. This chart will give you a score if any of the observations are out of target range. Once you have got your score, it will give you an explanation of how often to do observations and when to refer to the crisis team/doctor. However, as I said, always use your own clinical judgement alongside this assessment. If a patient doesn't look well, you seek help and further review of the patient (Royal College of Physicians, 2017).

SEPSIS 6 Pathway: This is a flow chart that you can find on the Sepsis website. If any of your observations are out of range, start to think 'is this potentially sepsis' – does the patient have an infection? Are they well? Are their observations out of range? Start the sepsis pathway and BUFFALO (below) if the answer is yes to these.

SEPSIS: If you suspect sepsis in any patients – Think BUFFALO.

B = Blood cultures

U = Urine output measurements

F = Fluids/give IV fluids

A = Antibiotics

L = Lactate measurements

O = Oxygen

Waterlow Score: This is an assessment which assesses a person's risk of developing pressure sores/ulcers.

This assessment considers: gender, age, build, appetite, skin conditions, mobility, continence, any long-term conditions, smoking, neurological deficit, surgery and medications. It will then calculate a score based on these.

Scoring: under 10 – lower risk

10+ at risk

15+ high risk

20+ very high risk

Depending on the score will depend on what you do next, start regular pressure relief for example.

I hope this chapter has given you everything you need to start your placements, good luck!

FUN FACT

Walt Whitman a famous poet volunteered as a nurse during the civil war. His poem 'The Wound Dresser' is based on his personal experiences on the battlefield (The Waltz Whitman Archive, n.d.)

References

BAPEN. (n.d.) *Malnutrition universal screening tool* [pdf]. London: BAPEN. Retrieved from https://www.bapen.org.uk/pdfs/must/must_full.pdf. Accessed 1 June 2021.

British Geriatrics Society. (2017). *Deconditioning awareness*. Retrieved from https://www.bgs.org.uk/resources/deconditioning-awareness. Accessed 1 June 2021.

CQC. (2019). *2018 Adult inpatient survey: statistical release.* Retrieved from https://www. cqc.org.uk/sites/default/files/20190620_ip18_statisticalrelease.pdf. Accessed 2 January 2023.

Filson, K., Atherholt, C., Simoes, M., DiPalma, M., John, S., Reynolds, R., & McGovern, J. (2018). Post-operative vital signs: How often is too often? *Journal of Clinical Oncology: An American Society of Clinical Oncology Journal, 36*(30). Retrieved from https://ascopubs.org/doi/abs/10.1200/JCO.2018.36.30_suppl.210.

GCS. (2021). *The Glasgow structured approach to assessment of the Glasgow Coma Scale.* Retrieved from https://www.glasgowcomascale.org. Accessed 30 May 2021.

Hanson, A., & Haddad, L. M. (2020). *Nursing rights of medication administration.* Retrieved from https://www.ncbi.nlm.nih.gov/books/NBK560654/. Accessed 15 July 2021.

NHS. (2010). *Safer care: SBAR.* Retrieved from https://www.england.nhs.uk/improvement-hub/wp-content/uploads/sites/44/2017/11/SBAR-Implementation-and-Training-Guide.pdf. Accessed 17 May 2022.

NICE. (2014). *Pressure Ulcers: Prevention and management.* Retrieved from https://www. nice.org.uk/guidance/cg179/resources/pressure-ulcers-prevention-and-management-pdf-35109760631749. Accessed 2 January 2023.

NICE. (2016). *Healthcare-associated infections.* Retrieved from https://www.nice.org. uk/guidance/qs113/resources/healthcareassociated-infections-pdf-75545296430533. Accessed 2 January 2023.

NMC. (2019). *Standards for competence for registered nurses [pdf].* London: NMC. Retrieved from https://www.nmc.org.uk/globalassets/sitedocuments/standards/nmc-standards-for-competence-for-registered-nurses.pdf . Accessed 25 May 2021.

Resus. (2021) *The ABCDE approach.* Retrieved from https://www.resus.org.uk/library/abcde-approach. Accessed 24 May 2021.

Royal College of Nursing. (2021) *Student nurses.* Retrieved from https://www.rcn.org. uk/get-help/rcn-advice/student-nurses. Accessed 24 May 2021.

Royal College of Physicians. (2017). *National early warning score (NEWS2).* Retrieved from https://www.rcplondon.ac.uk/projects/outputs/national-early-warning-score-news-2. Accessed 27 May 2022.

Royal Pharmaceutical Society. (n.d.) *Professional guidance on the safe and secure handling of medicines.* [online] Available at: https://www.rpharms.com/recognition/setting-professional-standards/safe-and-secure-handling-of-medicines/professional-guidance-on-the-safe-and-secure-handling-of-medicines. Accessed 2 January 2023.

Sherwood Forest Hospitals. (2019). *Observations and escalations policy for adult inpatients.* Retrieved from https://www.sfh-tr.nhs.uk/media/8331/observations-and-escalation-policy-for-adult-in-patients.pdf. Accessed 27 May 2022.

Stroke Association. (2021). *State of the nation [pdf].* London: Stroke Association. Retrieved from https://www.stroke.org.uk/sites/default/files/state_of_the_nation_2017_final_1. pdf . Accessed 30 May 2021.

The Waltz Whitman Archive. (n.d.). *The wound dresser 1865.* Retrieved from https:// whitmanarchive.org/criticism/current/encyclopedia/entry_749.html. Accessed 30 May 2022.

Yellow Card Scheme. (2021). *Yellow card.* Retrieved from https://yellowcard.mhra.gov. uk . Accessed 18 September 2021.

CHAPTER 9

Surviving Your First Night Shift

My First Night Shift – Story Time

On the day, I woke up around 5:30 a.m. so that I could hopefully sleep later, before my shift. I spent all morning thinking about this night shift. Panicking, worrying and feeling very anxious about it. Night shifts aren't something I want to be doing at all. I'm no night owl. I love my sleep.

> *I don't know how I'll cope!*
> *Nope. Stop it. Positive thoughts. Happy ones!*

I ate breakfast, ironed my uniform, got my backpack together and prepared my food for the shift. At 12:45 p.m., I get into bed, cover my head with the duvet to block the light but leave a tiny gap to breathe haha.

I actually managed to sleep for 2 hours, but I woke up a couple of times. I finally woke up before my alarm, feeling more tired than I did before! Urghhh. I made my lunch, washed, did my hair and makeup, dressed and then was out the door to catch the 5:05 p.m. train to get me there in time for a 7:00 p.m. start (it was a LONG journey to every placement for me).

I arrive at 6:30 p.m. and have a coffee to stay awake. I felt like a zombie and the shift hadn't even started. Here's a breakdown of what I did on shift:

- 7:00 p.m. Hand over.
- 7:30 p.m. Assisted a patient to change after they had soiled their clothing.
- 8:00 p.m. Removed a cannula from a patient's arm.
- 8:30 p.m. Measured the urine and documented it. With the sample, I did a urine dipstick test to check for urine infections in the patient.
- 9:00 p.m. Repositioned patients who needed this. Checked and recorded observations (blood pressure, pulse, temperature, respiratory rate (resps) and O_2 levels) on patients.
- 9:30 p.m. Aspirated a patient (using a syringe to drain out mucous/fluid from her nose tube) and documented it.
- 10:30 p.m. Wrote on the handover list online anything that needs to be updated.
- 11:00 p.m. Completed all fluid balance charts for patients. Observation (Obs) again on my patient.
- 11:30 p.m. Checked all patient documents to see if they were up to date.
- 12:00 a.m. Obs on my patient again (some are done more regular if they have any abnormal results).

- 12:30 a.m. Cross-checked for anything I've missed to let my mentor know.
- 1:00 a.m. Assisted the healthcare assistant to change a patient and reposition them.
- 1:30 a.m. Checked fluid balance was up to date again, checked catheter bags.
- 2:00 to 3:00 a.m. Break time. Chill. Eat.
- 3:00 a.m. Obs again. 'I feel so tired!' I sat and ate food, and now I need sleep. 'Not long left. Come on!'
- 4:00 a.m. I seem to be wide awake again. More obs, assist a patient to the toilet.
- 4:30 a.m. Document notes. Check all fluid balance charts are up to date.
- 5:00 a.m. All patient obs this time. And reposition patients who need it.
- 6:00 a.m. My mentor says I can go early. 'Whooooo!'

As soon as I left and entered the daylight, I felt so tired. I felt the night shift take over me. 'I was JUST fine?!' It's amazing how the body works.

Overall, it seemed like a quiet night. In between patients, I managed to fill out my practice placement document and do a little revision for my physiology. Kept my mind occupied, I think. I was surprised at how fast the night actually went. I was expecting it to drag, and I'd clock watch and hate it all. But it was OK. I wasn't rushed off my feet, everything went as smoothly as it could. All patients were comfortable and safe (minus me disturbing them for their obs). I don't know what I was worried about after all. Pros and cons of my night:

Pros: Less busy, you can manage your time better and work steadier to look after each patient properly. Not that you don't care for patients properly, but compared to a day shift, it's less busy because people are mainly resting and sleeping. No visitors, etc., as well. I prepared myself really well for the night shift: plenty of sleep, food and fluids to keep me going; I only felt tired a couple of times for a moment, and then I was great.

Cons: I don't feel like I've had a life outside of the hospital. Work, sleep and back again. I have a long trip so makes the night even longer. My routine is all messed up. And if you have a partner who works during the day, you might not see each other as much if you work opposite shifts (which might be a bonus for some people).

It is a Nursing and Midwifery Council (NMC) requirement that student nurses experience the 24/7 healthcare system (NMC, 2018). This might mean night shifts, weekends and bank holidays. However, if you have a health condition that is affected by doing night shifts, there might be adjustments made for you. Discuss this with your occupational health department at the university.

Some people absolutely love night shifts, and others do not. From my own experience of night shifts, mine were very relaxed. It didn't seem as busy during the night, and I felt I had more time to breathe and care for patients. I took my placement documents to my shifts, and when it was very quiet, I sat and filled out my book and revised for my exams. It is the perfect time to catch up on these things. I personally didn't like night shifts, and I couldn't get used to them at all. After my third night in a row, I felt so sick and exhausted, but, again, not everyone will experience this.

MY BIGGEST TIPS FOR NIGHT SHIFTS

- The night before, either go to bed as you normally would or try to stay up as late as you can.
- The morning of the night shift, get up as early as you possibly can, I got up at 5:00 a.m. I did my normal daily chores, like washing, cleaning the house, and I had breakfast.
- Have a nap in the afternoon for a few hours before you leave. Black out your windows, use an eye mask, ear plugs or anything that will help you sleep. I slept at around 1:00 to 3:00 p.m.
- Make sure, during this sleep, your house is quiet – tell your family to let you sleep.
- Have dinner as you normally would but make it a lighter meal rather than a big, heavy one that is going to make you want to nap. Less carbohydrates and more energy foods, such as vegetables, fruit, nuts, salads.
- Take snacks with you to your placement for your breaks during the night. Avoid big meals, again, this is going to make you sleepy. Take snacks such as nuts, fruits, vegetables with humus rather than stodgy meals like pasta.
- Keep a water bottle filled to drink throughout the night – stay hydrated.
- If you're feeling rather sleepy and your patients are all safe and sound asleep, which they will be around 3:00 a.m. (I'm not sure why, but this seems to be the time that most people get overtired). Get up and walk around. Start cleaning, tidying your trollies etc. – anything to keep you awake.
- Avoid caffeine just before you finish your shift because you want to sleep when you're finished.
- When you finish, have some breakfast when you get home (that's just what I do, some people don't like to do this).
- Shower, wash, get those pyjamas on, get into bed and try to sleep.
- I managed to sleep through the day after my first night. I woke up around 3:00 p.m.!
- Once I woke up, I had some dinner and got ready for my next night shift.
- Eating healthy meals like salads and vegetables rather than meals like pasta, roast dinners, etc. will help you feel more refreshed for your night shift.

I hope this helps settle your nerves a little around nights and give you some tips to help you survive your first night – good luck, you got this!

Reference

NMC (2018) *Part 3: Standardsfor pre-registration nursing programmes* [pdf] London: NMC, Available at: https://www.nmc.org.uk/globalassets/sitedocuments/standards-of-proficiency/standards-for-pre-registration-nursing-programmes/programme-standards-nursing.pdf. Accessed 31 January 2023.

CHAPTER 10

Applying for Your First Newly Qualified Nurse Post and How to Decide Where to Work

Congratulations, You Passed All of University! But What Happens Next and How Long Does It Really Take to Get Your NMC Pin Registration?

I was January 2017 intake at university, so our course ran from January to December each year. Technically, I finished everything at the end of November 2019. I didn't have to make up any hours and I did not have any outstanding exams or assignments etc., thankfully. However, because the course runs through until December, our exam board wasn't until January 2020. This is the date you need to find out from your university to work out roughly when you'll get your classification and Nursing and Midwifery Council (NMC) emails. I can only assume they have regular exam board dates every month. And my next assumption is, whatever month you started is when yours will be. But I'm not 100% certain so don't take my word for that one. Double-check with your university. But if you're at Birmingham City University and January Intake, yours will be in January, unless they have changed this of course, which can happen with time.

Our exam board was on the 9th of January 2020, to be exact. We then got our official classifications uploaded online and sent by email (a generic email to inform you to look online), which happened 7 days later, on the 16th of January 2020. Then, 24 hours later, on the 17th of January 2020, I received my NMC email congratulating me and asking me to go online to fill out my registration and pay my fee. All in all, 8 days from the exam board! However, I do know that there were some students who still hadn't received their NMC emails for around 2 weeks. So, I would say overall it probably takes between 7 and 14 days from the exam board roughly to obtain your NMC PIN.

What Happens When You Apply for Your NMC Registration? (It Took Me Around 10 Minutes Maximum to Do This – But I Am a Fast Typer)

Firstly, you have up to 6 months to apply for your NMC registration once you get your email invite. Some people take some time out of nursing before applying for their PIN, some people will travel abroad, for example. However, if it's over 6 months by the time you apply to register and get your PIN, there are some extra bits, you'll need to do. You will need to provide the NMC with a reference from a registered nurse or midwife, which is a supporting declaration. For them to be able to do this, they need to have

- Known you for a minimum of 1 year
- Been in regular contact with you over the last 6 months
- And they need to be able to confirm your declaration (NMC, 2020a)

The NMC will send you an email to your university email address which will provide you with the link to register. This is an automatic email that everyone will receive. In this email, you will also receive your NMC PIN at the top (clearly written and you'll need this to log in).

You will get to the first page which has the option to log in or register – You will click on register as you are registering. On the second page, you have to insert your name, email and PIN to get you logged in and started. This will then set up an account for you with the NMC, and this is what you'll use for the rest of your nursing career (unless they change it). They will then email you a link to verify your email, and then you will be officially signed up. Once you've signed up, you will have some questions to answer like:

- Are you in good health to practice?
- Do you have criminal convictions to declare?
- Have you been up for fitness to practice?
- Ethnicity
- Sexuality, religion and how you identify

Once you've gone through these, it will take you to your payment screen, where you have your annual fee of £120 (NMC, 2020b) to pay (prices correct as of 2020, which may change over time). There are options to pay quarterly or annually online. I choose to pay annually (I had to put this on my credit card because I was so poor then!) However, some trusts will pay your fee for you, which is lovely. So, check this out before you go ahead and pay this.

Once you've paid, that's it! You wait for your last email to say you're on the register! I had my email within 2 HOURS! Fast service or what?! And I can honestly say that it's possibly the best feeling in the world receiving that email. I can only imagine this is what winning the lottery feels like. All my journey has been totally worth every second for that moment in time.

Nurses are a unique kind. They have this insatiable need to care for others, which is both their greatest strength and fatal flaw.

JEAN WATSON, American nurse theorist and nursing professor

Applying for Your First Newly Qualified Nurse Job

It's the most nerve-wracking time but also the most exciting part about qualifying. For me, I knew where I wanted to work. After I had my second-year placement in a General Practice (GP) surgery, that is where I aimed for, and that's where I looked coming to the end of my degree. But how do you pick if you have no idea where you want to work? Think about what you have done already, where did you enjoy, or where did you not enjoy – erase it from your list: process of elimination. What sort of things have interested you during your nursing degree? That will be a good start. You can also start to make a list, what clinical skills did you enjoy using on placements? What type of human body system are you most interested in? What sort of hours do you want to work? This will help narrow things down too.

However, if you can't decide, some trusts do a rotational preceptorship where you will spend a few months in an area, then move on to another area. This is a good way to get more exposure to different areas you may not have experienced yet. Another way you could do it is by joining the trust's bank team or an agency to go to different areas. A 'trusts bank team' are staff who are not permanent to that area, and just do hours as and when they want to across different areas of one trust. So, for example, I was bank staff at a hospital in Birmingham, I could pick the days and hours I wanted to work at any ward I wanted to work on as and when I wanted to.

There are so many different areas you can work in, it's hard to narrow it down to just a few to apply for. But the good news is, the world always needs nurses, you won't be out of a job any time soon. And if you don't enjoy a workplace, you can move on. There's no harm, in swapping roles and areas, if you are not happy. At the end of the day, this is your career, and we spend most of our lives at work, so it's important to love what we do.

There are so many job sites out there to choose from, use them all! Most of the sites will ask for some sort of supporting statement or personal statement when applying for a nursing role. This is your time to shine and show how you meet all the essential criteria for their post. In your personal/supporting statement, you want to put your experience with examples of how you meet these. Below are my top tips for your personal statement (Box 10.1). Disclaimer, these are purely tips I use to help me, it's YOU that has to write it and get yourself that interview, no one else. Make use of your university careers team and the Royal College of Nursing (RCN) careers team (if you are a member) to help you.

Different Roles in Nursing

The beauty about nursing is, you can do anything, go anywhere in the world and there is always a high demand for nurses. Not only that, but the variety of nursing out there. However, there are so many roles out there and it's hard to cover all of them; university will only teach you so much, the rest is up to you to do your research. Which is why I am adding some extra stuff here for you. A little bit to get you thinking about alternate roles out there that you may never have thought of and may want to pursue in future. So, in no particular order, here are some of my favourite finds:

BOX 10.1 ■ Tips for Your Personal Statement

1. Write it on a Word document first and get someone to proofread it before you copy and paste it into the job site application form.
2. Copy and paste the essential criteria from the job specification onto a Word document, and use these as subheadings to structure your statement. BUT remove the subheadings before submitting your statement.
3. Use examples when answering the criteria of how you have met these as a student/nurse.
4. Regardless of how much or little experience you have, you will have so many transferable skills for the role. Make a list of skills you have that could be transferable and use them in your statement.
5. Don't repeat yourself – don't add anything that they already know from your application, such as education and employment. You will have documented this already; this is your time to show your skills and how you meet the role.
6. Don't waffle, keep it simple, straight to the point, and show that passion for nursing.
7. Make your statement specific to the trust or area you are applying to; include what it is that you love about the area you're applying to and why you are applying.
8. Use the STAR technique (situation, task, action, and result) to explain with your examples.
9. Using skills such as teamwork and how you do this, using your own initiative, different communications skills you have, any nursing assessments you may have used, and any you have done.
10. Make your statement stand out from all the others – use personal goals and achievements, something you have done that you are proud of. Anything that is going to sell yourself but also make you stand out.

SEXUAL HEALTH NURSE

An amazing role! I worked in sexual health for almost 6 years as a healthcare assistant. It's such an interesting and rewarding role. This is a list of the things that our clinics did and some of the things you might be doing in this role (list not limited to and different clinics may do different roles) are:

- History taking
- Care planning and concise documentation
- Health promotion and advice on sexual health and contraception
- Track and trace (that's right, this was a thing way before COVID-19 happened!)
- Swabs from different areas of the body, including genitals
- Taking blood for viral load testing such as human immunodeficiency virus (HIV) and hepatitis
- Giving treatments such as contraception, antibiotics, nitrogen treatment, creams and antiviral medications.
- You could be trained to insert implants and coils for contraception
- Training and education within schools and services

- Seeing a whole variety of patients from all fields of nursing and a variety of ages too
- Dealing with sensitive information
- Dealing with traumatic events such as sexual assault

SCHOOL NURSE

These are nurses who care for children, young people and their families. They aim to help reduce inequality and support and protect vulnerable children whilst improving their health. For this role, you will need specific qualifications after university called **Specialist community public health nurses.** School nurses will also work all year round, not just during school hours. They also work in collaboration with other people, such as community nurses, social services, nursery nurses, GPs, health visitors etc., to enable them to give the best care possible. Some of the things they do day to day are:

- Holistic assessments
- Safeguarding
- Relationship, sex and health education in schools
- Support to young people and families
- Supporting children with a variety of complex needs or long-term health conditions
- Equipping and empowering children to make better life choices and teaching them to access healthcare settings (National Health Service (NHS, n.d.).

NURSE LECTURER

Another amazing role and something I often think about doing at some point. As a nurse lecturer you are responsible for creating and delivering high-quality educational materials to students. You could work within a school, college or university, and some of your roles will include (list not limited to):

- Designing course material
- Marking work: assignments, exams, OSCEs etc.
- Being a personal tutor and academic assessor for students
- Answering queries, taking part in extra-curricular activities, teaching
- Meeting NMC criteria and standards for courses

(Royal College of Nursing, 2019).

CRUISE SHIP NURSING

'Say whaaaat?' You heard this right; you can become a cruise ship nurse and travel the world. I hadn't even thought about this until I saw someone on social media doing it and sharing their journey. I was quite surprised at the level of equipment they have on board too which can include x-ray machines! I know!? Wow. Who would have thought? Not me. With this, you do need specific training within the emergency department or Intensive Care Unit, between 2 and 3 years before applying for the level of autonomy you need onboard. Anyway, through some research around this role, some of the things you can be expected to do are:

- Provide healthcare and acute care
- Emergency support to travellers
- Safety onboard
- Documenting
- Good balance as you'll be on a ship which is a little wobbly…
- First aid
- Wound management
- Medications management
- Equipment checks

(Cruise Ship Nurse Jobs, 2019).

NASA NURSE!!

That's right the National Aeronautics and Space Administration (NASA) needs nurses too – I hadn't even realised this was a thing, but of course it is, why wouldn't NASA need nurses? Haha. So, these nurses are specifically for the NASA space centre and their staff/astronauts. As you may imagine (or not) being an astronaut comes with great risks to your health, and they are exposed to extreme environments which may damage their health. Some of the roles involved are:

- Health advice and promotion
- Giving treatments and medications
- Doing observations and physical examinations
- Screening for diseases
- Completing assessments and documentation
- Long-term conditions (such as diabetes and cardiovascular disease) care and even palliative care of patients
- Mental health assessments and treatments/advice
- Infection control
- Critical care and first aid

(Pandian et al., 2021).

AIR AMBULANCE NURSE

This is another role that really excites me thinking about it. I have watched air ambulance on TV and thought it must be such an incredible feeling getting that call out to a critical situation. Not knowing what you will go into and what you will have to handle at the time. Some of the things you would do in this role are:

- Attend emergency situations
- Give lifesaving treatments
- Anaesthetic or emergency medicine (depending on qualifications)
- Dealing with trauma
- Recusation procedures

- Medical interventions on ground and in the air
- Delivering pre-operation medicines

(Air Ambulance, 2022).

AMBULANCE NURSE/NURSE PARAMEDIC

If you're looking at working in the ambulance without completing the para-medic course and maintaining your nurse title, then this is for you. I would have enjoyed this role, I think, but I really don't like working nights or bank holidays etc. (personal preference). Some of the roles you will be doing here are:

- Treatments
- First aid
- Life support
- Asses, treat and manage different conditions
- Pre-hospital emergency treatments and duties
- Trying to avoid admissions to hospitals
- Dealing with major accidents and emergencies
- Treat, discharge and transfer patients
- Assessments
- Documentations
- Drug storage and equipment/drug checks
- Driving responsibilities

(NHS Jobs, 2022).

PRISON NURSE/CUSTODY NURSE

A prison nurse is very similar to a GP nurse. Type of things you might do here is:

- Safeguarding
- Minor injuries/illness
- Palliative care pathway
- Dealing with alcohol or substance misuse
- Mental health assessments
- Giving medications and treatments

(NHS, n.d).

- Custody nurse: Fit to detail examinations
- Medications
- Emergency treatment and situations
- Forensic samples
- Giving advice to police and prison departments

(CRG, 2020).

ABORTION CLINIC NURSE

There's a lot of debate in the news about abortions, but whatever your beliefs or views on this, it is still needed. And as nurses, we should never judge any of our patients and provide the best care we can to each person. This role can be very rewarding for the right person and some of the duties may include:

- Testing: Pregnancy tests, venepuncture, and results of these
- Ultrasound scans
- Giving health advice and information
- History taking and confidentiality
- Discussing treatment options with patients
- Ensuring informed consent is gained
- Sexually transmitted infection (STI) testing and contraception advice and treatments
- Administration
- Explaining different care pathways
- Mental health and physical assessments and reviews
- Post-operative care

(Bpas, n.d.)

FORENSIC NURSE

As a forensic nurse, you help care for victims of crime. You will be collecting a variety of evidence and samples. Some duties include the following:

- Care to victims
- Assessing victims
- Taking swab samples from victims
- Speaking with family, friends and law enforcements
- Assisting the families of the deceased people

(Indeed, 2021).

RETAIL NURSE (SUPERMARKETS HAVE THESE)

This is something else I had never thought about. But if you think about any supermarkets with healthcare inside, such as Superdrug or Boots, they all need a nurse. This is a nice way to do more sociable hours too. Things you will do here are:

- Consultations
- History taking
- Assessments and reviews
- Vaccines
- Blood tests
- Observations
- Following Patient Group Directives (PGDs)
- Health promotion

(Superdrug, 2022).

TV/MOVIE NURSE

These nurses can either advise television (TV) sets on different medical conditions and how they present them to enable actors to do the best job they can in the role they are playing. Or they can be nurses who tend to crew and actors in an acute emergency or injury situation. For example, if someone was doing a dangerous stunt and was injured. The nurse would go in to assess the situation (Nurse Organization, 2022).

CARE HOME NURSE

As I have discussed, I used to be a care assistant. I absolutely love the nurse's role in care homes. You will do shift work here, possibly nights, weekends and bank holidays too, because care work is a 24-hour service. Here is a list of things I have seen whilst working in care homes from the nursing teams (this is based on what our homes used to do and may vary from home to home):

- Assessing patients
- Observations
- Care planning
- Giving medications
- Working with GP's and other community teams with the patient
- Catheter care
- Pressure ulcer care
- Wound management
- Fluid and diet charting and assessing
- IV giving
- Palliative and end-of-life care
- Updating records and patient documents
- Risk assessments
- Personal hygiene
- Percutaneous endoscopic gastrostomy (PEG) tube feeds

I hope this section has given you plenty of food for thought! There is so much variety in nursing, so have a look around and see what you can do next. Some of these roles do expect experience and further training to be able to be competent at the role, so make sure you check all the necessary requirements before applying.

FUN FACT

About 40% of nurses do not work in a hospital (ECPI, 2022).

References

Air Ambulance. (2022). *Clinical recruitment & Selection*. Retrieved from https://theai-rambulanceservice.org.uk/our-work/work-with-us/join-our-medical-crew/. Accessed 20 May 2022.

Bpas. (n.d.). *Job requirements*. Retrieved from https://www.bpas.org/media/1520/nurse-midwife-practitioner-occ008.pdf. Accessed 20 May 2022.

CRG. (2020). *What is it like to work as a custody nurse? – Jo's story*. Retrieved from https://crg.uk.com/crg-medical-services/custody-nurse-interview-jo-davies-story/. Accessed 20 May 2022.

Cruise Ship Nurse Jobs. (2019). *Ship nurse job requirements*. Retrieved from https://www.cruiseshipjob.com/nurse-jobs.html. Accessed 20 May 2022.

ECPI. (2022). *What percentage of nurses work in hospitals: where else could I work?* Retrieved from https://www.ecpi.edu/blog/what-percentage-of-nurses-work-in-hospitals-where-else-could-i-work-as-a-nurse. Accessed 16 May 2022.

Indeed. (2021). *How to become a forensic nurse: A step-by-step guide*. Retrieved from https://uk.indeed.com/career-advice/finding-a-job/how-to-become-a-forensic-nurse. Accessed 20 May 2022.

NHS. (n.d.). *School nurse*. Retrieved from https://www.healthcareers.nhs.uk/explore-roles/public-health/roles-public-health/school-nurse/school-nurse. Accessed 20 May 2022.

NHS Jobs. (2022). *Ambulance nurse*. Retrieved from https://www.jobs.nhs.uk/xi/vacancy/917038759. Accessed 20 May 2022.

NMC. (2020a). *Register as a nurse or midwife if you trained in the UK*. Retrieved from https://www.nmc.org.uk/registration/joining-the-register/register-nurse-midwife/trained-in-the-uk/. Accessed 25 May 2021.

NMC. (2020b). *Register as a nurse or midwife if you trained in the UK*. Retrieved from https://www.nmc.org.uk/registration/joining-the-register/register-nurse-midwife/trained-in-the-uk/. Accessed 25 May 2021.

Nurse Organization. (2022). *The glamourous side of healthcare: Hollywood nurses*. Retrieved from https://nurse.org/articles/hollywood-nurse/. Accessed 20 May 2022.

Pandian, V., Coker, D., & Shelhamer, M. (2021). Nursing care in space – the need for nurses in the new and evolving field of healthcare in space. *Journal of Clinical Nursing, 31*(1–2). https://doi.org/10.1111/jocn.16092.

Royal College of Nursing. (2019). *When the student becomes the teacher*. Retrieved from https://www.rcn.org.uk/magazines/students/2019/when-the-student-becomes-the-teacher. Accessed 11 May 2022.

Superdrug. (2022). *Popular services*. Retrieved from https://healthclinics.superdrug.com. Accessed 20 May 2022.

CHAPTER 11

CV Writing

A curriculum vitae (CV), what's that?! Yes, places do still ask for a CV. If you are applying for a general practice (GP) nurse position, for example, some clinics will require a CV application. So, I am going to give you all the advice I can for CV writing. Firstly, ask your university careers team to help you out. If you send them your CV, they can help edit it and give you pointers on how to improve. Next, if you are with the Royal College of Nursing (RCN), they have an RCN careers team to whome you can send your CV and ask for advice too. I used both teams to help with my CV application. But they will also help with personal/supporting statements too for work applications, so use them to your advantage; that's what they are there for. If you are writing a CV as a new university nursing graduate, your CV will be different from a regular one. You will be putting your recent 'nursing experience' from your placements instead of job list.

However, you can also add recent roles that you have had around university, but only if they are relevant to the role you are applying for. For example, health-care assistant work or volunteering for care homes/healthcare professional roles.

To get started, firstly, have a look online for CV templates to help you start, but here are the headings and layout I used, and this is my own exact CV template I use every time (Fig. 11.1).

Go onto the job you are applying for and use the person specification and job description to help write your CV for each role you're applying for. Use this to include the essential criteria needed for the role you are applying for. Then add them to show you have the right skills needed to fulfil the role. I usually do mine on a Word document first, I write subheadings of the 'essential criteria needed for the role', and then under the subheadings I will list my skills and experience so far. Once complete, I then copy and paste the relevant information across to the CV. The CV needs to target the trust/company you're applying for. Adjust each CV to the place you're applying to so that it makes it personal to them. You can also have a generic CV that you can keep ready to submit anywhere, but a more personalised one will show them you are motivated and interested in them.

At the top of the CV, you want your personal information so they can contact you. Personal information should include your name, address, email, phone number and website/social media (if you want to, this is not essential, it's just what I do so they can go and see all the things I have been doing out there). I add all of this at the top of the page and then use my name as the 'Title' of the CV. I used to write Curriculum Vitae (CV) as the title, but I was advised this is not a good look

Miss Claire Carmichael
Email | Mobile
Address:
Twitter / websites: @CCarmichael_83 | LinkedIn Account

Professional Profile:

A little bit about you and your work ethic, passion, ambitions

Key Skills and Achievements

Add your skills and achievements here such as: communication, assessment planning, things such as IV, bloods, catheters etc.

Nursing Experience:

Birmingham City University, Birmingham.
- ADD YOUR PLACEMENT SKILLS HERE USING SHORT BULLET POINTS

General practice (12th March 2018 – 30th April 2018)
- Skills gained: ADD YOUR SKILLS HERE

District Nursing (2nd September 2019 – 22nd November 2019)
Community Rehabilitation ward (25th March 2019 – 27th May 2019)
Stroke ward (21st August 2017 – 30th October 2017)
Abdominal surgical ward (27th March 2017 – 22nd May 2017)

Healthcare Assistant (Band 2). Sexual health (March 2014 – December 2019)

Care Assistant for the elderly Residential home (August 2013 - October 2013)

Care Assistant for the elderly Nursing home (December 2010 - October 2012)

Extra-Curricular Activities / Nursing Experience:

Ambassador - General Practice Student Nurse Network - NHS England (October 2018 – present)

Ambassador - The Academy of Fabulous Stuff NHS (September 2018 – Present)

International student's mentor - Birmingham City University (August 2018 – August 2018)

High Achievers Recognition Scheme Scholar - Birmingham City University (Feb 2018 – November 2019)

Education:

BSc (Hons) Adult Nursing Birmingham City University – First Class Honors January 2017 – January 2020

Access to HE Diploma with **English level 3** and **Numeracy level 2** (Sept 2011 - July 2012)
   Passed with 57 credits at level 3 (Distinctions and Merits) and 3 credits at level 2.

City and Guilds Numeracy and Literacy level 2 – passed (Learn direct 2001)

GSCE's, (September 1999 – July 2000)
   Art, French, English, Maths, Science, Music and Food Technology.

References available

Fig. 11.1 Sample CV template.

and is not professional, and to keep it as your name and details instead. Once you have added your personal information, the next subheading you want is 'Personal profile'. In this section, you want to write no more than a couple of sentences. This section should include what you're doing now, your skills and experience for that role and what you are now seeking. For example: '*I am a newly qualified nurse (third-year student nurse) with experience as a GP nurse ambassador and previously had a placement within GP and fell in love and now seeking a long fulfilling career as a GP nurse*'. You could even add your future goals, advanced nurse practitioner etc. if you wanted to show your long-term plans with them.

After this section, you want a 'Skills' section and within this part, you should give a list of the skills you are competent in, such as venepuncture, observations,

---

BOX 11.1 ■ What Not to Add to Your CV

- Don't add 'Curriculum Vitae/CV' as your heading at the top (use your name instead).
- Don't list every single job you have had – it's not needed.
- Don't write anything that isn't related to the role you're applying for.
- Don't tell them your life story. Don't add training and skills that are not relevant to the role.
- Don't repeat yourself.
- Don't waffle.

IT, communication, catheter care/insertion/removals, wound management, suture/clip removals, vaccines and injections, electrocardiogram (ECG), anything you have been signed off to do. Again, with this part, read the person's specification to show you meet their criteria for the post. You want to be ticking all their boxes for this position throughout the CV.

The next section is the 'Education' part. This is where you list any qualifications and schools/universities you have been to, from General Certification of Secondary Education (GCSEs) to your university degree details. Keep it brief and simple.

Following this section, you add your 'Nursing experience' heading. Where you list all nursing-relevant experience, placements, volunteering and anything relevant to the post you are applying for. For student nurses, I listed my placements here and what I learnt (clinical skills included) on each one.

After this, you can add any work experience. This is where I added my paid employment here, things such as healthcare assistant work, I had done over the last few years. You can add just a brief role description, places you worked and dates to and from. Keep it brief and simple again. I only added nursing-related roles here; anything else not relevant and any gaps in employment, I added as a sentence below.

I also worked in hospitality as a waitress, receptionist and housekeeper from 2001 to 2005.

Purely because they aren't relevant to the role I am applying to, but the placements and care home experience is. This helps to keep the word count down too. You can also add an 'Achievements' section. If you have done anything extra, such as won an award in or outside of university. Any achievements you have gained that you are proud of to show your dedication and work ethic. Don't be shy to celebrate your small or large wins in life. Unlike a standard application form, you don't need to add references. You can add a small section at the end of the CV that says 'References', and you can write 'references available on request' to save space and word count. If successful for the job, they will then ask you for references later. There are some mistakes I have made before with my CV, so I wanted to add a 'what not to add to your CV' and break it down for you to help you out (Box 11.1).

Constant attention by a good nurse may be just as important as a major operation by a surgeon.

—DAG HAMMARSKJÖLD, Swedish Economist and Diplomat

CHAPTER 12

Transition from Student to Newly Qualified Nurse (NQN)

I must be completely honest with you here; the transition from student to qualified nurse was by far the hardest part of my nursing journey. No one prepared me for this, university couldn't have prepared me for this feeling and nothing I write here will prepare you for that moment either.

When you qualify it's very exciting with a mix of nerves. You're starting your new job; you're taking your first selfie in your uniform and posting it online because you finally made it! Then, your first pay comes along, and you're deciding what you're going to spend it on. However, all of that goes a little downhill if you don't have a good support network. I'm not talking about your own family this time, I'm talking about your work family and your old university friends etc. Those people who truly understand what it's like to be a nurse and can give good advice when you need it.

As a newly qualified general practice (GP) nurse, it can be very lonely and isolating, and this support network is needed more than ever! I say this because that was me. Not only had I started working at the beginning of a pandemic, but I had also moved area and I had no friends, I was starting a new workplace, it was exciting, but I didn't realise how lonely it would feel. I've always thrived on my autonomy, and I didn't ever expect to feel this kind of feeling. I hit, quite possibly the lowest I have ever felt in my entire life. I started to question whether I made the right decision coming into this career. I wondered if I should have gone to another area instead. I was going home crying a lot and just felt like utter rubbish. My mental health had gone from thriving to diving…

If it wasn't for the amazing support from my General Practice Nurse Student and Nurse Network (GPNSNN) team, I don't think I'd have coped. Making connections with other GP nurses and newly qualified GP nurses really does make all the difference! It's so lovely to talk about what's going on and how you're feeling. We have our WhatsApp group where we can sit and chat and go over our days, or we will discuss things in our virtual meetings. It's nice to know there is someone to turn to when I need it most. I'm usually that person for everyone else, so it's hard to realise when I need to help myself. I was also put in touch with another newly qualified nurse who was feeling all the same things as me; it was lovely to be able to support one another.

The next thing that really helped me was being part of the fellowship programme. The fellowship programme is a new programme available in some parts of the UK (not all parts sadly). It is a 2-year 'preceptorship' type of thing; you get funding for training and extra support to help you transition into a GP nurse. Part of the programme is that you get put onto the fundamentals course through university, which is a specific course to train you to be a GP nurse. This course is only available to those working as a GP nurses, as you have to get your competencies signed off in clinic with a mentor.

Sadly, my fundamentals course (which is part of the fellowship) was postponed due to COVID, so I was now 8 months in as a newly qualified nurse (NQN) and I was just starting it. I then had a whole class of around 20 NQNs or nurses new to GP, and they all felt the same way. I felt like I had a good, strong group of nurses who would all support one another, and it was fabulous! I also made friends with another nurse on the course who is in the same boat as me; just moved area, new job and have no friends or family locally! I wonder if I had started this course at the beginning like I should have, I'd have felt better from the start. I think so.

And lastly, friendships. I recently met one of my lovely social media buddies, who lived not far from me. We met up for some socially distancing tea (because it was still during the pandemic) and cake, as well as a good natter about life. It wasn't until I got home that I realised how much I needed that. She may have saved the last piece of my sanity without realising it, haha!

It's times like this, I think back to my training and what I learnt along the way. I remember the talk about 'Maslow's Hierarchy of Needs', and if one of the needs is taken away, it can really affect a person (Fig. 12.1).

A section of mine was taken away from me: 'love and belonging' – I no longer had friends around me or a sense of connection/belonging. Furthermore, evidence shows that when this is taken away, your health and well-being suffer as a consequence (Hale et al., 2018). However, it's important to look at everyone individually and holistically to see what the bigger picture is and other factors that contribute to this.

Nevertheless, one of my needs had been removed which resulted in the others being chipped away at too. 'Self-actualisation' – I was finally a nurse, after 12 years and setbacks along the way. I was here and I felt that I was failing… I felt not good enough, so my 'esteem' went down with it. As a result, what was I left with? I was surviving on 'physiological needs' and 'safety needs.' I was the captain of the Titanic that hit the iceberg, and I was slowly going down with the ship. It's no wonder I felt so low and struggled with all of that going on. As I reflect today, I'm proud that I got through that. But so grateful for the people around me who helped get me through those times.

And lastly, if I can feel like this then anyone can! I'm the most motivated and positive person you'll meet, and it affected me. How many others are feeling like this? How many people have left the nursing profession because of it? What things are in place to help NQNs out there? Do they have a good preceptorship?

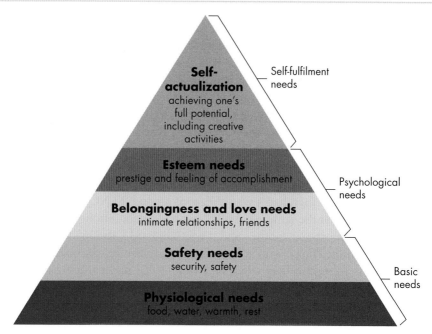

Fig. 12.1 Maslow's Hierarchy of Needs. (Image sourced from McLeod, S. (2007) *Maslow's hierarchy of needs. Simply psychology*. Retrieved from https://www.simply-psychology.org/maslow.html. Accessed 30 May 2022.)

Is it good enough? Now I'm left with more questions and wondering how can this be improved?

Therefore, it's so important to get support if you're struggling. At the start I kept hearing:

> *'It's ok, it's normal to feel overwhelmed as a newly qualified nurse' and 'it can take up to a year to settle in'.*

But is this 'normal' and is this OK? Because no, this isn't OK, and nurses shouldn't be feeling like this. We should be thriving and keeping that passion alive. So, absolutely, more needs to be done to help NQNs out there. So, wherever you are working, whether you're a student or a newly qualified nurse, please get support if you need it. Please don't just go with it and start to run on empty. YOU are just as important as your patients. You have to be the best you can be to be able to care for others effectively.

Story Time

When I first started my GP nurse post, I had a patient in my clinic for some blood tests. The patient asked me 'what does it mean when your potassium is too low?'

I had no idea; my mind had gone blank. I beat myself up a lot over this and kept thinking, 'I have just done a 3-year degree, why don't I know this?!' This added to my low confidence and self-esteem, as discussed. But after the patient left, when I had some spare time, I sat and did research on the types of blood and what different ones did in the body. So, if anyone else asked me, I would have the answer next time. I still have this all written down that I keep in my drawer today – luckily, I haven't needed it again!

But the real answer is, even the top consultants don't know it all. No one can physically know it all, so please be kind to yourself. Nursing is a huge area, with so many different specialities, different conditions, different medications, different medical presentations, it's quite easy to get lost in it all and feel like 'Alice: Lost in Wonderland'. And lastly, if you're applying for a role, ask the question in your interview, 'what support will be put in place for me?'. If they don't satisfy that answer, then keep looking. Because a good manager will have things in place to support their staff already.

Always remember, you're worth more, you ARE capable, you CAN do this. Keep being you and don't go down with the ship – instead, sail to the shore towards the sunrise.

Tips for the transition phase:

1. Take your time, this isn't a race.
2. Don't compare yourself to other NQNs.
3. Get more training; nursing is lifelong learning.
4. Make sure you are well supported by your team.
5. Ask for support if you need it.
6. Remind yourself you can't physically know it all.
7. If you are unconfident with something – ask for more training on this.
8. Do research around the subject you aren't familiar with.
9. If you aren't well-supported and feel unhappy in your first role, don't be afraid to find somewhere more supportive.
10. Make sure you stay connected with your friends and family for extra support.
11. And lastly, if your team are not supporting you after you have asked for advice and support, you're entitled to find somewhere that is supportive. Don't be afraid to change roles or the workplace. Ask for an exit interview when you leave so that you can give constructive criticism and they can improve from this.

FUN FACT

The nursing exam that foreign nurses take in Japan is so difficult that only 94 out of 741 have passed it in the last 5 years (pre-2013). It consists of 240 questions, and it is 7 hours long! (Today, 2013).

References

Hale, A. J., Ricotta, D. N., Freed, J., Smith, C. C., & Huang, G. C. (2018). Adapting Maslow's hierarchy of needs as a framework for resident wellness. *Teaching and Learning in Medicine, 31*(1), 109–118. doi:10.1080/10401334.2018.1456928.

Today. (2013). Japan sets high bar for foreign nurses. Retrieved from https://www.todayonline.com/world/asia/japan-sets-high-bar-for-foreign-nurses. Accessed 30 May 2022.

CHAPTER 13

Nursing Interviews

Congratulations!! You have bagged yourself that first nurse interview! A huge well done! But what to expect? In this section, I am going to give my best advice on my own experiences as well as hear other newly qualified nurses' (NQNs) experiences of their interviews.

I have had a total of five interviews which I will go through now with you.

1. **Community Nurse Band 5 Post.** For this interview, I had two people in the room asking me questions: A human resource (HR) person and the lead nurse. They made me feel at ease and like I had known them for years! It was lovely. Some things to think about during this interview include things such as:
   - What skills can you bring?
   - You arrive at a patient's house, and they are on their way out for lunch. What do you do?
   - Explain what Integrated Care Teams are and how they benefit patients?
   - You are in charge of the shift, and you have three new calls in: (1) End-of-Life (EOL) medications, (2) A wound that wasn't done yesterday and (3) A blocked catheter. Which ones do you prioritise and why?
   - What checks would you do for an EOL patient on a syringe driver?
   - Can you think of EOL paperwork/assessments?
   - If you witnessed a staff member being unsafe, what would you do?
   - How would you handle loan work?
   - What risk assessments are there for the community?
   - If you found a patient had a pressure ulcer, what would you do?

2. **3 × GP nursing post interviews.** Another interview that I had had two interviewees: the practice manager and a GP nurse. I was made to feel so welcome and part of the team before I even started. These interviews (I had three different practices and all similar) were very relaxed and more of a general talk than anything else. Some things to think about in this type of interview are:
   - Transferable skills you might have such as ECGs, wound management, communication, injection technique, long-term conditions you have seen, sexual health and contraception, suture and clip removals after surgery, observations (blood pressure, heart rate, temperature, respiratory rate).
   - Mental health referrals – who's your local team?
   - Quality Outcomes Framework (QOF) and how GPs get funded.

- Working autonomously – how will you cope? Think about scenarios: angry patients, how you'll handle this alone?
- What is a Primary Care Network?
- What skills can you bring to a team?

3. **Education trainer in a hospital.** This was a great post I applied for and got the job! I turned it down in the end though, as I was offered something else that was going to give me a better work-life balance to be able to finish this book and other things, I was setting up. For this interview, I had a couple of nurses and a nurse manager interview me. They were really lovely and made me feel so welcome. If you are going for this kind of role, some things to think about for the interview are:

- Any training, teaching, education you have done yourself for students, nursing teams etc.
- KNOW THE TRUST VALUES and know them well! Nine times out of 10, if I have applied to any NHS trust, they will always ask you what their values are and how you will implement them. So, check them out and give examples.
- Know the area you will be working, what they do, the role, and have a good understanding of what's expected of you. Because they do usually ask what you know about the role.
- Again, you might have some scenarios based around educating others, types of learning styles maybe?
- How to handle a complex situation, such as safeguarding concerns, if they arise.
- How to manage language barriers and different communication styles
- How you will help students/nurses to strive to be their best self
- Any ideas or things you have put in place in practice to help with education?

All interviews will have their standard type of questions they ask such as

- Tell us about yourself?
- What skills do you have to bring to the team?
- Where do you see yourself in 5 years time/what are your ambitions?
- Why do you want to work here? Or be a nurse here?
- What experience do you have in this role?
- What do you know about this area/trust/ward etc.?

You may have some scenarios such as

- If you had an angry patient/relative, how would you cope with the situation?
- If you made a drug error, what would you do?
- If one of your colleagues was doing something wrong, what would you do?

As previously discussed, I get so overwhelmed by interviews, and this really knocks my confidence on the day. I end up underselling myself and not saying the things I could be saying to make them want me.

Story Time

In fact, in my very first interview, I messed up hugely. I was moving from Birmingham to Portsmouth, and I didn't know the Portsmouth area well at all. I was so nervous that when they asked me which town I was moving to, I replied with 'Pompey' because I thought that was the name of the town, I was going to be living in… I had no idea it was a slag word for Portsmouth haha whoops! Luckily, they found this hilarious, laughed at me, and told me what it meant – and offered me a job anyway. Sometimes these little mess-ups break the ice and make you likeable, so don't be worried if this happens to you. Laugh it off, apologise and keep going!

However, my last few interviews have gone very well! I have managed to hold my nerves together and am able to sell myself as best as I could for each of the above.

It can be hard to overcome nerves, but just remember this is just as much as their interview to you and you are to them. You might have several places to choose from, and they will have to sell themselves as well, this is a two-way street. There is always that one question at the end that no one ever knows how to reply: 'Do you have any questions for us?' Yes, yes you do! You just didn't realise it. You could ask them a variety of questions about the role, the team and how they work, but one question I really love is, 'What do you love most about working here?' I think this is a great question to see what it is. Another great question are, 'How will you support me as a newly qualified nurse?' Because you want to make sure you are well supported, like we spoke about in the transition section. Some other questions you could ask is, 'What training packages do you do for newly qualified nurses' or if you really don't want to ask anything, you could say 'I was going to ask about such and such, but you have covered that for me, thank you.' That's a line I use if I really can't think of anything to ask them. Just never forget to sell yourself well, because that could be the one thing that helps you get that post. I know this from my many failures at interviews, and all the feedback is always 'you didn't sell yourself enough'. So, please, put all your fears aside and go get it! **Good luck everyone!**

> ***FUN FACT***
>
> Knights who fought during the crusades become nurses. They enjoyed it so much that they took on the nurse role permanently and were called Knight Hospitallers (Nurse Buff, 2018).

Reference

Nurse Buff. (2018). *Fun Facts you probably didn't know about nursing*. Retrieved from https://www.nursebuff.com/facts-about-nursing/. Accessed 30 May 2022.

CHAPTER 14

Maths/Drug Calculations Made Easy

One of the other most popular questions I see out there is this one. Student nurses seem to fear maths, I feared maths. The drug calculations exam was the one thing I dreaded alongside the dissertation. My maths was shocking, and in fact, first-year exams were the hardest for me! First-year maths at my university was all about fractions, decimal places and equations. I *just* scrapped passed this with a 7/10, which was the pass rate for this year. I made stupid errors like putting the decimal in the wrong place or adding a 0 by mistake. I discovered I was far better at working out real-life scenarios in the second and third years with real drug calculations. Please, do not panic, you may not understand it right now, but you will. Like with everything in life, practice makes perfect. The more you can do to practice doing online tests, revision, learning the techniques to solve the equations, you will be way more confident at it.

Firstly, I am awful at maths – I got mainly Ds and Es in my General Certificate of Secondary Education (GSCEs), so this is why I was so anxious. But if I can do this, you *can* do this! I have faith in you. However, if you suffer from any type of learning need, such as dyscalculia (a maths learning disability), please contact your university and inform them so extra measures can be put in place for you to help you.

When you apply to university, you *may* have to sit a maths and English exam before being interviewed. Please do not panic over this! Not everyone will have these exams either. These exams are very basic, honestly. For the maths, it is multiplication, division, subtraction, fractions, decimal place and percentages. This exam is just basic level 2 maths, and it will be the same sort of exam in your first year too.

Next, second year, we hit the drug calculations. This exam I was worrying about this more because I thought it would be a lot more complicated than it was. But if you read the question, use the equation to work it out, you will be fine. For our university we were given a calculator, which made a huge difference.

So here are a couple of questions you may get:

- Doctor prescribes 5 mg of a medication, and you have 10 mg in 2 mL in stock. How many millilitres will you give the patient?
- A patient weighs 69 kg on arrival to your ward. But when they are discharged, they weigh 57 kg. How much of a percentage of the weight has the patient lost?

- A medication is prescribed as 0.2 g daily, to be given in two equally divided doses. State in milligrams the amount of drug needed for each individual dose.
- The doctor has prescribed 100 mg of prednisolone in 1000 mL to be given in IV over 30 minutes. How many millilitres per hour should the pump rate be set at?

The first one is quite easy, I think. What do you think? Doctor prescribes 5 mg, and you have 10 mg in 2 mL. The answer to this one is literally just half of what you have = 1 mL. Because there is 10 mg in 2 mL, so there is 5 mg in 1 mL. If that makes sense. Your answer is 1 mL. BUT if you have a different lot of numbers and you are unsure, there is an equation that will help you out here (Box 14.1). What you need/what you have × by the volume.

The next question is about finding the percentage of body weight lost. And there is an equation for this one too. Firstly, you want to see how much body weight has been lost, so using the details, in the equation below we can try and work out someone's body weight loss. Say you have someone who is now 57 kg, but previously they were 69 kg. So, their weight loss in kg is 12 kg. Because 69 − 57 = 12. Now you want to use this 12 kg in your equation.

$$\text{Weight loss/Original weight} \times 100$$

Now you use this equation to work it out as a percentage. 12 kilograms (weight loss) divided by 69 kg (original weight) and then multiply by 100 to get the percentage = 17.3913043 (what your calculator will show). Because you have a decimal place, you need to round this one up or down to get a whole number (your university will tell you to round up or down, so only do this if told to do so). Anything below .4 so, .4, .3, .2, .1 is to be rounded down. Anything above .5, .6, .7, .8, .9 is to be rounded up. So, in this example, we are rounding it down to 17% because it is 17.3913043. So, the answer is 17% weight loss.

The next question can be a bit trickier; Doctor prescribes 0.2 g daily, to be given in two equally divided doses. State the amount of drug in milligrams. You can do this one a couple of ways: The first way is you can convert it into milligram to start with (Box 14.2).

Lastly, the IV pump rates. I think this question, again, is simple, but have a look and see what you think.

BOX 14.1 ▪ Drug Calculation 1

You take what the doctor has prescribed you (the 5 mg), divide this by what stock you have got already (the 10 mg) and then multiply this by your stock volume (2 mL – the millilitres it comes in). So, no matter what numbers you get for this question, you have the right equation to work this out easily.

So, this would be: 5/10 = 0.5 then × 2 = 1 mL.

BOX 14.2 ■ Drug Calculation 2

To convert gram to milligram you multiply by 1000. If you were to go from milligram to gram you would divide by 1000.

In this example, we will do 0.2 g × 1000 = 200 mg. Now you can work out the rest. It asks for two equally divided doses, so literally 200 divided by 2 = 100 mg (the answer).

The other way you could do this is to work it out in grams first and then convert to milligrams at the end. For example, 0.2 g divided by 2 = 0.1 g. Then change it to milligram, so 0.1 × 1000 = 100 mg. Whichever is easier to understand for you, use that.

You have your 100 mg in 1000 mL already for 30 minutes. But you need an hour, so you are literally just multiplying by 2. Because there are two lots of 30 minutes in 1 hour. The answer is 2000 mL over an hour. However, you may get a trickier question like, you have 100 mg in 1000 mL set over 40 minutes. How many millilitres per hour do you set the pump rate at? For this, firstly, get your answer per minute.

1000 mL divided by 40 minutes = 25 mL (per minute)

Now you have the millilitres per minute you can multiply by 60 as you need this set over an hour. 25 mL × 60 minutes = 1500 mL/h.

And that is it. I really hope this helps you to understand these calculations a little bit better. I am the sort of person who needs a simple, layman terms explanation, and I hope I have managed that here for you all. There are a few websites to help you with drug calculations, such as the Royal College of Nursing drug calculations page, but again, please speak to your university and see if there are any extra tuition sessions available for you if you need more help with these. I know our university gave us lots of practice papers to do online as well which really helped. Hopefully your university does this too!

Routes of Drug Administration (Box 14.3)
HOW DO MEDICATIONS/DRUGS WORK IN THE BODY?

Medications have a chemical reaction in the body: the drug will combine with your body chemicals to either create a reaction or neutralise something. For example, medications for acid reflux work by neutralising the acid in the stomach.

Some have a physical effect on the body, such as osmotic (a process where liquid is drawn through a solid barrier). They draw water from your body into your bowels to soften your faeces/stools (poo).

Enzyme inhibition = A medication that stops/reduces an enzyme in the body.

BOX 14.3 ■ Medication Abbreviations

Oral	By mouth: tablets/liquid/capsules
Sublingual or buccal	Either under the tongue or between the gum and cheek.
Transdermal	Through the skin via a patch
Topical	Onto the surface of the skin such as creams.
Ocular	Into/onto the eye
Nasally	Into the nose
Inhalation	Inhaled into the respiratory system, such as inhalers for asthma
Subcutaneous (Subcut)	Under the skin
Intramuscular (IM)	Into the muscle
Intravenous (IV)	Into the vein
Rectally (PR)	Into the rectum
Vaginally	Inserted into the vagina

Ion channel blockade = Blocks ion channels, such as medications like amlodipine, which work by blocking the channels which then causes vasodilation (widens blood vessels) and reduces blood pressure.

Fitting into receptors = Most drugs do this and either block the receptor they bind to or cause stimulation to increase production. Drug receptors sit on the outside or inside of the cells.

Agonist = I always think this as 'aggravate', that's the way that helped me remember that it stimulates the receptor/cells to get a response. Agonist = 'aggravate' something to get a response.

Antagonist = I always saw this as the opposite 'anti/anta' agonist. Like anti = anti aggravate. So, if it is the opposite of the above, it will block the receptor to get no response (Richards, 2014).

Something I wanted to add here is some science bits. Because something that we were taught, I really struggled to interpret into my brain, and I finally just got it one day. The difference between vasodilation and vasoconstriction and why it increases or decreases blood pressure.

Vasodilation = When the blood vessels in the body expand, they widen to allow an easier flow of blood through them. Now, when you initially think of this, you would think it causes blood pressure to increase, but it doesn't; it does the opposite. This reduces blood pressure when it does this.

Vasoconstriction = When the blood vessels narrow, they tighten up which means blood is being forced through them more because of the restriction. This increases blood pressure when it does this.

If you think about, think about a water hose, if you had a standard garden water hose, the water flows freely out of it. However, if you were to place your finger half way across the hole and the end of the hose where the water comes out (to make a smaller hole for the water to get through), the water pressure increases, and it appears to be coming out quicker than usual because you have restricted it, which means the pressure of this is higher. Or another way to think of it, is your shower. You can adjust the shower head to make the pressure of water higher or lower when it comes out of it. It's similar to blood pressure. So, if you think of your veins/arteries etc., tightening, closing, narrowing, the blood is being forced out at a faster pressure. But when they are widened, the blood can flow at a nice regular pace. I hope that explanation makes more sense to you and helps you understand how it works.

Never give up on a dream just because of the time it will take to accomplish it. The time will pass anyway.

EARL NIGHTINGALE, American radio speaker and author

Reference

Richards, S. (2014). *Nursing & health: Drugs in use* (2nd ed., pp. 3–15). New York: Routledge.

CHAPTER 15

Leadership in Nursing

The Nursing and Midwifery Council (NMC, 2019) 'Standards for competence for registered nurses' states that 'All nurses must: "act as change agents and provide leadership through quality improvement and service development to enhance people's wellbeing and experiences of healthcare."'

Before I started my nursing journey, I would never in a million years of thought I could be a leader and provide leadership to others. Especially after those General Certification of Secondary Education (GSCE) grades I got! When I thought about leaders, I thought of big, powerful, manager-type people. However, I was wrong, here I am writing this book hoping to create a better future for students and newly qualified nurses. What I have learnt on this journey, is that everyone can be a leader and you are probably already doing it whilst reading this book. I think of leaders in the same category as role models:

Role model: Noun. a person that you admire and try to copy. We need positive role models for young women to aspire to. Parents are a child's primary role models.
OXFORD DICTIONARY (2021)

I see leadership as encouraging others to be their best self and enabling others to see their own potential. Leading by example so that others will lead with you, not for you, not against you, not behind you, but right next to you or ahead of you. And that's what we all do realistically, in everyday life without realising it. When is the last time you commented on someone's social media post, encouraging them, or motivating them? When is the last time you guided your child for the best (if you have children)? When is the last time a friend came to you for advice? All these small things show leadership in some way. And we must be good leaders for our patients as nurses. We lead by example; we give health promotion to our patients and build that rapport so that they follow our guidance. If there was something that could be done better at work, you would encourage change in a way. If there was a skill you were performing which hurt your back, for example, you would find a better way to do this so that it stopped hurting your back, right? All great leadership skills.

People often think to be a change agent or leader, you must be bossy and tell people what to do. That's not it. And people often confuse management skills with leadership skills, but the difference is:

Leadership is about motivating people to comprehend and believe in the vision you set for the company and to work with you on achieving your goals.

While management is more about administering the work and ensuring the day-to-day activities are getting done as they should.

NEXT GENERATION (2020)

There are many books and guides around leadership, but the best thing you can do is do what you love and share that passion with everyone around you. My best tips I can give are:

- Not only share your achievements with everyone around you, but also share your downfalls and how you have overcome them
- Encourage and motivate others to be their best self
- If you haven't got anything nice to say, don't say it and never make a promise you can't keep (From my nan herself, the best leader and role model I had)

Be more self-aware and more aware of your emotions – emotional intelligence: Emotional Intelligence:

Noun – The capacity to be aware of, control and express one's emotions, and to handle interpersonal relationships judiciously and empathetically

Emotional intelligence is the key to both personal and professional success

LEXICO (2021)

- Share your ideas and new ways of working with your colleagues
- Share other people's success as well as your own
- Share things that work well in your area
- Take some time out for yourself (a tip I will regularly share with you). You must be your best self to be able to help others
- Listen and communicate effectively with those around you
- Be more human – you are not a robot, and it is ok to show this

Story Time

It was as a student nurse when I realised that you could lead and be a huge influencer at any level of nursing – you don't have to be senior or qualified. This leadership journey of mine started in the second year of my nursing degree as a student. But what happened to start this journey? How does someone become a leader? Can leadership be taught? In my opinion, leadership is within us, we all have it deep down somewhere, it's just learning how to bring it to the surface to help others. And some people might not want to do that. Gardenier et al. (2020) states, 'Not everyone can or wants to be a leader, but if you are a nurse, it simply comes with the territory. Ensuring that we have effective leadership qualities and skills is a way that we ensure we will continue to meet the needs of our patients and society'. However, there are ways that we can be taught in leadership skills. Something such as Insights Discovery sessions, which included leadership, coaching and mentoring others as part of the High Achievers Recognition Scheme through my university, Birmingham City University (BCU). The first skill I learnt was all about myself. I had completed a profiling form which then was analysed, and this created a whole profile about my personality, strengths, weaknesses and how I can use them to the best of my ability. But also, how to work with people who are the opposite to me: Which is definitely needed in healthcare. I say this as there are many different personality types out there, and you might clash with some of them. It's important that we recognise this and work professionally with these opposites for the best outcomes for our patients.

Completing this sort of profiling for yourself can really help with your emotional intelligence and recognise your weaknesses and how to overcome this. It's the first step to good leadership, I think (again, just my own opinion here. It's ok to disagree with this).

- *But this would be my first tip to leadership: Complete a self-discovery profile*

Anyway, back on track, during my second year, I started my General Practice (GP) placement and fell in love with it. So much I had to write blogs and do vlogs all about it and share it with the world and whoever would listen. I soon discovered that people were listening to my passion, people I never thought would ever speak to me. It was like a ripple effect across social media! Have you ever seen the dancing man video? Let me explain: There's a field, with lots of people sitting on the grass in separate groups. The sun is shining and there is music playing. One man, on his own, stands up and starts to dance. He's having a great time on his own, dancing to the rhythm of the music, so much so, another person gets up and starts dancing too. The two start to dance and look so happy, so then, another person stands up and starts dancing too until the whole field of people are up dancing and having fun. This is the ripple effect. I connected with so many nurses out there, some of whom had been qualified for years and messaged me to thank me for bringing the positivity and love of nursing back to them! I had inspired people I had never met; I had encouraged people into nursing, into GP nursing too! And then, I had an inbox from a nurse leader, asking if I would attend and do a talk at a GP Nursing conference with them. I was so shocked! I was terrified of public speaking, but I also wanted to push myself, so I agreed to do it.

I was then sat in front of a room full of GPs and nurses from across the country, talking about my journey and how we needed student nurse placements out there (we still need more placements). I do have a funny story to add here.

Story Time - (*continued from a previous chapter*)

During my first talk at the conference, I had worn odd socks under my trousers that day. In my head, I thought I would be standing so no one would see them. And then I was faced with a chair to sit down on to do my talk… I had two options: 1. Don't mention it and hopefully no one will notice; or 2. Mention it and point it out (something my introvert self would never do). I chose the second option.

> *"I just wanted to say sorry to you all, I have odd socks today, I didn't realise I would be sat down, and people would see these haha"*

I chose to point them out and use this as my ice-breaker talking point. Which seemed to go down well with people.

I was then invited to another conference to talk about leadership at all levels, during which someone said this was the first time a student nurse has stood and talked about this during a conference. Don't get me wrong, I was terrified! I was never a public speaker before; I was very introverted (and still am), and that was my comfort zone. However, if you stay in your comfort zone, you don't grow. Someone once told me, 'To be able to speak, do vlogs, put yourself out there, you have to forget what people think of you'. And it was true – the moment I stopped thinking, 'gosh, who will see this video, or who will judge me for this' I felt more relaxed.

> ■ *So, my second advice to you is: Forget about what other people think of you and step outside of your comfort zone. You have nothing to lose, but a lot to gain from it.*

Now, I am going to backtrack slightly – sorry folks. Back to my first year of the nursing degree. We had a university event called 'staying successful' at around 6 months into the degree. A halfway point to say, 'you're doing amazing, keep going' and some options for societies and extra-curricular things to do around university (uni) life. I had started university, I just wanted to get my head down and I just wanted to pass the course and qualify. Until this moment, this was my 'light bulb' moment.

Light Bulb Moment

Noun: a moment when you suddenly realise something or have a good idea:

It was a light-bulb moment for me when I realised I could no longer go on without help.

CAMBRIDGE DICTIONARY (2021)

There was a fantastic speaker, Dave Keeling, who was not only a comedian but a motivational speaker too and the one thing he said, was my moment: 'Do you want to go through the next 3 years of university and regret not doing enough?' 'Do you want, to just get your head down, work hard, pass exams, then you're qualified but then look back and think, I wish I did more at uni?'

He was right; I was that person. I was the one wanting to get my head down and just pass. He spoke right into my soul and changed my life that day, and I have never been the same since. I decided to start looking into societies; I started the High Achievers Recognition Scheme (HARS) work-shops at uni; I started tweeting on Twitter and then I picked up a camera and I started vlogging and blogging. And that was the start of my leader-ship journey, the stepping stones that then pathed my way to GP nursing and more.

- *So, my third tip for leadership: Don't bury your head and just get by – get out there and do more. This is genuinely what has kept me motivated during my career, doing more, and helping others.*
  - Every single person will have their own leadership style because we are all different and unique. This is your superpower: no one is you. Find what works for you and what doesn't, and grow from there.
  - Don't compare yourself to other people; you are not them, and they are not you
  - Listen and learn from others
  - If someone gives you advice, take it, listen and improve

Here Is a Lovely Section on Leadership By a Third-Year Birmingham City University Student Nurse Called Felicia Ikponmwosa

You know, going along in this course, I've had an experience of good and I have had an experience of the bad. But with the determination and resilience, I have been able to get this far.

Now, when I started as a first-year student. Everything seemed rosy, every-thing was going on smoothly. We started our first-year placements, and the knowledge wasn't there, and the confidence was not there. The skies were sup-posed to be light. And before you know it, because we came and the pandemic came, boom, we were asked to stay at home. Took out of our nursing placements and we're at home until we were asked to go back. It wasn't every one of us that went back either. I was among those who could not, because it was affecting my mental health. I saw myself missing out on a lot. My colleagues were on place-ments, and I had to stay at home. But I helped myself, and I was using the period to study and plan on my coursework. So, the 5 weeks that I missed on placement passed, and we started our classwork again.

The second-year placements? My mental health in all of this remained affected and I saw myself missing out, not learning anything, not knowing any clinical skill. Then, when it was time for us to go for the third-year placement, the hospital to a very different world. A unique world where I became in charge. I became in charge because we were three third-year students. And there were the first-year students, and then there were second-year students, all on the same ward. There were so many that they divided us into two groups. So, your two third-year students were in one group, and I was alone in my group. I thought to myself, 'how will I, am I able to cope with this? Will I be able to cope in leading others?'

However, I found some qualities that I didn't even know I had. They were all in me, so I was really in charge, and I guess I played that role of a leader to other students.

What is it to be a leader? Being a leader, you have to be a role model for other people. I was able to do all of those things. I'm being a leader as a student nurse. I was able to even delegate. Delegation is crucial in leadership. Because at one point, my supervisor was telling me, 'Yes, you are doing well in your leadership role. However, I've not seen you delegating'. To delegate, in fact, it takes boldness to be able to delegate. Because you wouldn't know if you're going to offend people. You are delegating duties too. You would have support from the colleague and from my co-students. I was compassionate. I took their motivation, their knowledge into account in all these things that I was doing.

With other multidisciplinary team (MDT), for you to be able to deliver quality, care and safe care to patients. I took their motivation, their knowledge into account in all. So, as it is now, I have my confidence back.

So, we need to be able to take the knocks. We need to be able to problem solve, and you've sort of blossomed almost before your time.

> ***FUN FACT***
>
> In 1878, Calamity Jane nursed victims in the smallpox epidemic dressed as a man. She dressed and acted like a man and did mostly jobs men would do (Legends of America, 2019).

References

Cambridge Dictionary. (2021). *Light bulb moment.* Retrieved from https://dictionary.cambridge.org/dictionary/english/light-bulb-moment. Accessed 14 June 2021.

Gardenier, D., Szanton, S., & McBride, A. (2020). Can leadership be taught? *Journal for Nurse Practitioners, 16*(6), 414–415. https://doi.org/10.1016/j.nurpra.2020.03.003.

Legends of America. (2019). *Calamity Jane – Rowdy woman.* Retrieved from https://www.legendsofamerica.com/we-calamityjane/. Accessed 30 May 2022.

Lexico. (2021). *Emotional intelligence.* https://www.lexico.com/definition/emotional_intelligence. Accessed 7 June 2021.

Next Generation. (2020). *The difference between leadership and management.* Retrieved from https://www.nextgeneration.ie/blog/2018/03/the-difference-between-leadership-and-management. Accessed 7 June 2021.

NMC. (2019). *Standards for competence for registered nurses* [pdf]. London, UK: NMC. Retrieved from https://www.nmc.org.uk/globalassets/sitedocuments/standards/nmc-standards-for-competence-for-registered-nurses.pdf. Accessed 25 May 2021.

Oxford Dictionary. (2021). *Role model.* Retrieved from https://www.oxfordlearnersdictionaries.com/definition/american_english/role-model. Accessed 7 June 2021.

CHAPTER 16

Mental Health/Coping with Failures

Firstly, how are you? Kindness costs absolutely nothing and to some people, it might mean the whole world. One simple act of kindness can really make someone's day. Not only that, but you don't know what someone may be going through, and that last piece of kindness could really change things around for someone. I was told a story once, many years ago, I *think* it was at school… but I have to share it here. Warning: This story may trigger some uncomfortable responses due to the sensitive nature of the subject and talks of suicide. Please feel free to skip past the story (you will see a quote starting with 'I do love my job' where you can continue to read on from there). But I am sharing as this is the story that made me think about always giving kindness no matter how bad my own day has been. It's a story I think about every time I come into contact with another person, and it has really helped me be patient and kind to others when others may not have been kind to me.

Story Time

The waitress and the accountant. (Warning again: Talks of suicide in this section – please skip this part if you feel uncomfortable.) Story below is not a real-life story; however, it can happen.

There was a man called Dave, a 38-year-old accountant. He had just finished his long day in the office. His day has been awful, in fact; customers haven't been happy with him, and he's in need of a good drink in the bar to gather his thoughts before he goes home to his family.

Dave enters a restaurant/bar. Where a waitress called Laura tends to Dave. Laura is a 35-year-old waitress, she's just found out her boyfriend has been cheating on her, she's been fighting with her mum and has been struggling with her mental health a lot lately. However, Laura, on the outside, appears happy, smiling and laughing. She loves her job, it's her safe place right now; it's where she can go and forget about her home life and escape for a short while. Dave orders his drink from Laura and takes a seat in the corner. Laura brings over his drink; however, it was the wrong drink and Dave gets very angry about this. He's had a bad day at work and he just wanted a drink, so he swears at Laura and calls her incompetent at her job and that she needs training or even better… sacking!

Laura is so apologetic but Dave storms out and back home to his family. Laura is left feeling deflated, thinking 'he's right, I am an awful waitress' – this was the last straw for her. Her world was crumbling around her, and she couldn't take any more. She's lost her boyfriend, her mum and now she feels like a failure at her job. Later that night, Laura took her own life. Dave was the last nail in her coffin.

Now, let's take a back step, reverse time and go back to that moment when Dave enters the bar, orders his drink and sits down. Dave has realised he has been given the wrong drink. However, this time, he's aware of his own emotions and the fact he is having a bad day. He goes up to Laura and says 'I'm so sorry, but I think I may have someone else's drink, it's not your fault at all so please don't worry' – with a smile at Laura. Laura apologises and gets him his correct order. Dave finishes his beverage and leaves, leaving a tip for Laura on the table. Laura picks this tip up and smiles. She thinks to herself:

I do love my job; I think I'm going to apply for that management position I always wanted. And when I return home, I'm going to make a means with my mother and boyfriend.

Dave's, simple act of kindness has turned Laura's day and thoughts around. Can you see how the way you treat people with or without kindness really matters? This happens in real life. Someone will be struggling daily with battles you don't see on the outside. Their bucket is filling drop by drop with emotions, and what you say to that person, could be the last drop that tips the bucket over the edge and spills.

Please, despite your bad day, always be kind to others, as you never know what someone else is going through. I fully understand that sometimes it will take a whole lot more than a simple act of kindness to help people with a mental health crisis, but I wanted to give an example of how kindness can help others. Even if it's not everyone, your one act of kindness could potentially save someone's life.

Remember, you matter! Your health, whether it is physical or mental health, is so important. YOU are just as important as any of your patients, colleagues, friends, or family members. So, here are a few tips from my heart to your heart if you find yourself struggling right now:

- Meditation – Meditation helps to reduce stress, anxiety, helps lengthen attention span, improves sleep and much more (Healthline, 2020). There are so many free apps for National Health Service (NHS) workers right now too, so have a look. I have found this so beneficial for myself and I hope it helps you too. You can also search online for 'guided medication' which helped me keep calm during the stress of exams and assignments.
- Breathing techniques – These help to steady your breathing and heart rate and regulate that 'fight or flight' response going on right now. Breathing techniques are amazing because you can do them anywhere at any time you need them. Start with a simple one: breathe in through your nose for 1 to 5 seconds and then out through your mouth counting 1 to 5 seconds again. I usually do 4 seconds in, pause for 2 seconds and then 4 seconds out

slowly. Then repeat this for 3 to 5 minutes and hopefully you should start to feel a reduction in that anxiety you might be feeling (NHS, 2018)

- Getting outside – Talking a long walk, cycle, run, or some light exercise can help too. Although some days you may just want to hide under a duvet and cry it out all day, and that's ok too. Do what's best for you.
- Listening to music – Music is great for relaxation and calming the mind. I have recently discovered 8D music! It's music that you need your head-phones on for or it just doesn't work. The sound and vibrations of the song hit differently to your ears and make it a more immersive experience (Infographics Archive, 2021). I personally love this and use it when I feel overwhelmed. So, put your headphones on, search for 8D music, turn your favourite song up loud and enjoy!
- Hobbies/crafts – If you don't have or do any of these, maybe it's time to find something that you can fall in love with. I have started doing rock painting, clay making and resin art! It's so therapeutic to me. Or maybe you could learn a new language or how to play an instrument? Pick something for YOU, that doesn't involve nursing to take time out for yourself to relax.
- Therapy – This could be professionally, or just having a colleague, friend or family listening to you. It's so important to talk about your feelings, be open and honest. Even if you want to write it all down, get it out! Even if you don't know what to write, just get a pen/pencil, and some paper, and write… anything… whatever comes to mind, just start. And once you're done, tear it apart, like you're getting rid of all those feelings. It's better to get them out of your mind than lock it up and avoid it. You may cause yourself more harm in the future by doing this.
- Also, trying alternate therapies such as Lavender on pulse points really helps too! It's not for everyone and caution must be taken if you have aller-gies etc. But research has shown it can help keep you calm without the sedation effect of some medications (Malcom & Tallian, 2018). However, these therapies must never be used as an 'instead of' solution. Seek medical advice from your doctor/nurse before stopping any of your medications. I love lavender, I use it in my baths and on my pulse points before sleeping.

This list is not limited to, everyone is individual and what works for me may not work for you. It's about finding out what works for you and doing more of that. Everyone will handle their emotions differently and a mental health crisis will look very different in different people, so it's important to recognise the signs in yourself and seek help and advice where needed. And remember, you're not alone in this, there are people out there that will listen and help you. There is a light ahead of you, despite not being able to see it right now, you will be ok, and hopefully things will get better for you.

So, I will ask again 'how are you really?'

Nursing is tough! No one ever prepares you for it. You have placements, exams, assignments, revision, poster presentations, skills sessions, and anything else in-between. Don't beat yourself up if you get a low grade, or you don't pass something the first time. It's ok, and a grade or lesson learnt doesn't make you a failure. Once you qualify, all employers want to see is that you have that Nursing and Midwifery Council (NMC) PIN to be a registered nurse. And the best nurses I know didn't get great grades, and some don't even have a degree, they were the old diploma nurses. Because back in the day, you didn't need a degree to become a nurse. So please, do not beat yourself up and please be kinder to yourself. You have done/and are doing amazing!

MY TOP TIPS FOR FACING FAILURES ARE

- Take some time out to relax
- Read through any feedback you have on the assignment/exams/placements
- If you don't have much feedback – ask for more. I did this a few times: I emailed my marker and asked for more detailed feedback and they gave me quite a bit back which I could work on to improve in future. I also do this with job interviews too
- Also, sometimes there's a technology failure. If your feedback doesn't match your mark, email and confirm you have the correct mark, a few people I know (including myself) had this happen to them. I had an assignment back and the grade didn't match the feedback at all! So, I emailed the marker to see if something had gone wrong and it had. They had accidentally attached the wrong students' feedback to my assignment, and I actually had a higher grade
- Remind yourself, how far you have come and look at what you have achieved so far
- Remind yourself, not everyone passes the first time and that's ok
- Take some time off social media around results day! Because looking at other people's grades and achievements can make you feel awful without realising it
- Try and push aside your doubts – your brain will lie to you. YOU ARE DOING FABULOUS! Keep going!

During your nursing journey, at some point, or many points your mental health may take a tumble for the worst. Your nursing journey is one big rollercoaster of emotions. It's important that you recognise the signs of a dip in your mental health early on and get the support and help you need, some signs may include:

- Agitated easily
- Low mood, upset or very tearful
- Low self-confidence or low self-esteem
- Poor sleep
- Tiredness even after a good night's sleep
- Forgetful

- A change in your appetite
- Avoiding social interactions
- Mood changes/feeling anxious

(Mind Charity, 2019).

People you can speak to are your family, friends, personal tutor, uni module lead, uni year lead, occupational health, and your doctor. Anyone you feel comfortable with. But please, never suffer in silence, get help, and take some time off if you need it! Your health is far more important right now and you can't give the best care to your patients if you aren't your best self. There's been a lot of research on burnout in nursing and how the effects of this can result in errors being made and patient safety being compromised (Montgomery et al., 2021) and therefore it is important to get help before it gets to that stage.

As discussed in the transition to the newly qualified nurse chapter, I have suffered from a decline in my own mental health. And this felt awful, it felt as though I was stuck inside a deep black hole with no escape. Most days, I wanted to stay in bed, but I had to get up and go to work so I didn't let anyone down (which would have made me feel worse). When I did get home, I changed into my pyjamas, didn't eat properly (a lot of takeaways actually) and couldn't even face doing the dishes. It was a never-ending cycle, not eating well, then feeling worse because I hadn't eaten well. This went on for a good few months until I finally asked for help from my own GP and went to discuss things with the local mental health teams and got some cognitive behavioural therapy (CBT) sessions to help me with this. They put it down to grieving for my old university life and big changes to my own personal life. Luckily, I got better and I'm in a far better place today than I was that year. Mental health can take control in all sorts of ways, it will present itself as something different in everyone. Along with this, your mental health isn't less severe than someone else's, just because the reasoning behind it or triggers are different. Mental health is still mental health regardless of what the trigger is, it doesn't make you any less important than the next person. I hear so many times 'well it's not as bad as so and so...' and that's not ok, please don't compare your life and health to others, you are just as important and your health matters just as much. It can be really hard to say out loud that we are struggling, because we are nurses and so used to looking after everyone else. When we are sick, we start to feel guilty and don't want to be a burden on anyone. But you need to speak up. Find someone you can talk to, friend, family, a stranger, anyone who you trust, and you want to talk to. The most important thing is that you get help and support before it controls your life. Never feel ashamed or too proud to get help, it's a very common thing and we all go through some form of mental health issues throughout our lives. Don't suffer in silence.

What to Do When You Have an Action Plan From Your Supervisor

I was very fortunate to never have this happen. But I did get some good advice from mentors and what they needed to see from me to be able to sign me off at the end of placement. Also, I have been a practice assessor for students, so I hope I can give some good advice to help you get through this if needed.

Firstly, every placement has to give you a chance to improve. So, this is why, halfway through every placement you should have an interview/meeting with your supervisor/assessor to see where you are at and if there's anything you need to improve on. If they are not doing this, they shouldn't be allowed to fail you. Because they have not gone through the correct process to help you improve. If this happens or has happened to you, please appeal this. Unless you have put another person in danger or gone against your NMC code of conduct… that's a different story. It depends on the situation and if you can appeal it.

If your mentor gives you advice on how to improve, listen to them. Take on board what you need to do and set yourself some SMART (Specific, Measurable, Attainable, Relevant and Time-bound) goals to action the points they have made. If you don't understand anything your supervisor /assessor has said, please ask for further information and how you can improve.

SMART GOALS

Research shows that using SMART goals increased adherence by up to 63% in nursing (Revello, 2014). Smart goals are set to help you set and achieve goals and help you professionally develop.

SPECIFIC

Set a specific goal you want to achieve. Make sure it's very specific which doesn't leave it open for interpretation. So, for example, 'I am going to write 100 words on my safeguarding assignment in 1 weeks time.' Some questions you can ask yourself to help make this more specific is:

What do you want to achieve, why do you want to achieve this, where, when and how will you do this?

MEASURABLE

To be effective, you have to be able to measure what you are doing. Have a clear milestone. For example, 'I am going to write 100 words on my safeguarding assignment within 7 days. Then check in 7 days if I have done this correctly.' You have a target date to measure whether you have written 100 words or not. You can use the word document word count to measure this number.

ATTAINABLE

Your goal should be within your reach. It should be a realistic goal and not one that is too ambitious. You know your limits after all ☺. Don't make it harder for yourself, or you won't achieve the goal.

RELEVANT

Set goals relevant to what you want to achieve and that are going to improve something in some way relevant to you and nursing. There's no point in setting a goal if it is just a tick box for you. Set something meaningful that you will gain from.

TIME-BOUND

Set yourself a time frame on when you are going to achieve this. Set a specific date and stick to that target. Then break it down piece by piece how you'll manage this. So, for example, finishing your assignment within 1 month. Breaking each section down, to do one section a week. This goes back to breaking it down so it's manageable and doable.

Using powerful words such as 'I am' and 'I will' rather than 'I could' or 'I want to' will really help set this goal. And this is the same when writing something such as a personal statement, or job application, avoiding negative words such as 'I feel' or 'I think' shows you are unconfident in what you are saying. But changing those phrases to 'I am', 'I have', 'I know' can really make a big impact (Nurse Choice, 2018).

And SMART goals are used in a variety of ways, you could use these to set goals in your personal life too if you wanted to. They are great, and transferable across tasks you need to complete whether nursing related or not.

Bullying/Harassment in Healthcare and How to Cope

I have added this section as I have seen a few students ask about this or speak about this across social media – which is shocking! No one should ever be bullied or harassed in healthcare; however, if this is happening/happens to you, I hope that I can give some sort of advice here on what to do and how to handle this situation. I am in no way trained or an expert in this area, but I hope I can give you something which might help you out if ever needed.

Firstly, gather your evidence. As always, in nursing, we always need evidence otherwise it's one word against another sadly! Keep a log, a diary of dates and times and what has happened along with who else was there (any witnesses). Save emails, messages, and screen shots as evidence also, with dates and times and the person.

Next, if you feel comfortable enough to speak to the person yourself and sort it out – do this. Just bring them to one side in private or have a witness present and then professionally tell them how you are being made to feel by their words or/and actions.

If you don't feel comfortable doing this or this doesn't help the situation, then you need to go higher up the chain of command – the matron/manager/sister in charge or even the chief executive of the trust. Bullying and harassment should NEVER be tolerated in nursing and this needs to stop, so you really need to be brave and speak up and hopefully make change wherever you are. If you speak up, it can make a change for future students and hopefully this won't happen again. Sometimes it only takes one person to speak up and the rest will follow…

STORY TIME

A few years ago, I was a healthcare assistant in a residential home for young adults with a variety of learning disabilities. We were due to have a new resident move into the home from another city, who had quite complex needs. To help ease their transition from the previous home to the new home I was appointed their lead care worker. With this, I had to visit each week for several weeks to shadow the staff at the home, meet the resident, and build a rapport with them. So that:

1. They had someone familiar whom they trusted in the home.
2. Someone understood their complex needs and how to manage them daily and train the other staff with this.
3. Someone could create care plans and documents on their preferences and step-by-step guides to help them.

Part of this, I had to video tape little activities to show how the staff manage certain areas such as eating, walking, taking their medications. There was written consent provided by the family for all of this and everything was done legally which will then help the resident. Each time I visited I would stay onsite, get up when they got up in the morning to observe personal hygiene, the way they manage this, breakfast times, medications, school days etc. I consented to sit in class to help them and observe this as well which was great! Throughout my time, I sat, made notes, videoed different parts, observed, interacted, and built a good rapport with the resident. However, one of the activities I witnessed and videoed made me feel extremely uncomfortable. What I was capturing was the resident being pinned down and forced into their medications, which I knew was not right. I asked at the time 'why do you have to do it this way' and their reply was purely 'he won't take it otherwise', there was nothing in place to say this is how he had to do it. I went back to my manager after seeing this and reported my concerns. I had captured it on video (with consent as explained) and showed her this. She was horrified as well by this behaviour and she then showed his parents to ask if this was right, and if there was a reason, they did it this way. However, the parents were just as shocked as us with this. In the end, we all had to give statements to the police with what we had witnessed! Which was terrifying! I did not want to get anyone into trouble or lose their jobs. However, it wasn't right what they were doing there, and it needed addressing to stop this from happening to anyone else in future. This meant, when the resident came into our home, we worked alongside the parents and doctors to have the resident's medications adjusted so that he could have them inside food, it was in liquid form, powder form, it was all adjusted and done properly to enable the resident to have their medications safely and without the need to restrain them. This is how this should have been done from day 1. And in doing this, we had no concerns at all with their medications and this was managed really well by everyone involved.

The point of my story is, sometimes you must speak up. No matter how afraid you might feel. And sometimes, your gut will tell you something is not right, follow your gut. If someone's actions or behaviour towards another person makes you uncomfortable, it's probably wrong and needs reporting. And even if you report it, and it is all ok in the end, it's far better to report your concerns, document it and be safe than sorry.

You have to think 'if they can do this to one person, how are they treating other people?' We have to protect others, as well as ourselves at the end of the day. However, I know how hard this can be, and the worry of any backlash from speaking up against staff. It's important you get support if you do speak up and ask to be kept anonymous if you fear what will happen to you as a result.

Nevertheless, if you really can't speak up yourself, some tips are:

1. Speak with your work, placement team or placement lead person
2. Tell your manager or placement team what is going on so they can support you
3. You could write an anonymous letter/statement of events and what's been happening and leave it on the manager's desk – this will then plant the seed and hopefully, they will put things in place to monitor this person or investigate the complaints made
4. You could get a union involved to help support you
5. Speak with colleagues, family or friends whom you trust about it (maintaining confidentiality of course).

Caring is the essence of nursing.

JEAN WATSON

References

Healthline. (2020). *12 science-based benefits of meditation*. Retrieved from https://www.healthline.com/nutrition/12-benefits-of-meditation. Accessed 10 May 2022.

Infographics. (2021). *Why ADHD and Neurodivergent people are into 8D audio*. Retrieved from https://www.infographicsarchive.com/why-adhd-and-neurodivergent-people-are-into-8d-audio/.

Malcolm., B. J., & Tallian, K (2018). Essential oil of lavender in anxiety disorders: ready for prime time? *Mental Health Clinician, 7*(4) Retrieved from doi: 10.9740%2Fmhc.2017.07.147.

Mind Charity. (2019). *Depression.* Retrieved from https://www.mind.org.uk/information-support/types-of-mental-health-problems/depression/symptoms/. Accessed 8 June 2021.

Montgomery, A. P., Azuero, A., Baernholdt, M., Loan, L. A., Miltner, R., Qu, H., et al. (2021). Nurse burnout predicts self-reported medication administration errors in acute Care hospitals. *Journal of Healthcare Quality*, 43(1). Retrieved from doi:10.1097/JHQ.0000000000000274.

National Health Service (NHS). (2018). *Breathing exercises for stress.* Retrieved from https://www.nhs.uk/mental-health/self-help/guides-tools-and-activities/breathing-exercises-for-stress/. Accessed 14 May 2022.

Nurse Choice. (2018). *Nursing Smart Goals: How to set smart goals for nursing.* Retrieved from https://www.nursechoice.com/blog/profiles-and-features/nursing-smart-goals-how-to-set-smart-goals-for-nursing/. Accessed 14 May 2022.

Revello, K. (2014). *An educational intervention to increase nurse adherence in eliciting patient daily goals.* Retrieved from https://onlinelibrary.wiley.com/doi/pdf/10.1002/rnj.201.

CHAPTER 17

Having Autism and Epilepsy – A Case Study from Sez Francis

I met Sez through the power of social media. I found her vlogs as I was searching for different health conditions to gain more knowledge as a student nurse. And what better way to learn, than through the patients themselves! I would sit and watch Sez's YouTube videos all about her autism, epilepsy and living her life. She raises so much awareness around these conditions, it's amazing and I have learnt so much. I asked Sez if she would write me a little piece to add to the book from her perspective, how she feels about her diagnosis. I really hope, this helps you all to understand it from a patient's perspective and gives you some food for thought when you are caring for those out on placements and when you qualify. My biggest tip – do research around the patient's perspective and their conditions, it's the real way to learn in my opinion. There's only much anatomy and physiology will take you, the rest is up to you. A huge thank you to Sez Francis for writing this. I absolutely owe you big time, the biggest reward is teaching others and creating change out there – Thank you (Box 17.1).

Sez Francis – Having Autism and Epilepsy – A Case Study

Sez Francis: '*If we move in together, would you help me in an emergency in case I have a seizure?*' This was what I asked my boyfriend while we were out together for lunch on one of our date days. Usually, I wouldn't ask that question to anyone outside my family; however, helping him to prepare for what to do if I have an epileptic seizure means a lot to me. Not just for when we take the next steps in our relationship together but when we are out and about too.

I worry about the *what-ifs* of me having a seizure or him supporting me when I'm panicking about some unexpected incident – in front of him and out in

---

BOX 17.1 ■ Epilepsy Description

Epilepsy: A condition that affects the brain. Someone with epilepsy can have different types of seizures, and these can vary in how often they occur depending on the person. A seizure is when the cells in the brain cause an intense electrical activity that causes a disruption (Epilepsy Action, 2021).

public. Luckily, I didn't have to practise the panicking part since he knew what to do when I'm upset. However – he has never seen me having a seizure!

I'm still dreading how he will react if that happens, but I try not to think about it too much.

However, it isn't just that; there are so many things I worry about:

- What'll happen if I am living on my own?
- What'll happen if I am living with another person instead of my parents?
- Will I receive **the support** I need?

And these are some of the questions you should be asking about your patients. You want to know they are well supported and be thinking holistically.

I do overreact in many situations and struggling to support myself is often the underlying cause (Box 17.2).

I was diagnosed with atypical autism and global developmental delay when I was 2 to 3 years old; but for the icing on the cake, I was also diagnosed of having a language disorder and a learning disability. I am a complicated person, let me tell you that!

I don't remember anything during my diagnosis process but when I was growing up, I would question myself: *why am I different?* and *why do I see these strange words on my medical and education documents?* Since I can remember, while my Mum and I would visit a General Practice (GP), I would distract myself by secretly reading over the doctor's notes while the experts and my parents were talking. I was inquisitive and I would self-question whilst trying to mask my emotions. I found it hard since I would feel nervous about my appointments, especially waiting for my turn in the waiting rooms. One time, my mum and I waited for nearly an hour and a half for an appointment; and it was like living in a butcher's shop. I know it won't make sense to you, but it does to me. This is how my mind works.

Different GP practices can be different for everyone, but my practice is relatively small, small like a crowded cabin lodge. When it's busy, there's no room to swing a cat. There's no room for a quiet space if there is a patient like me who is oversensitive to noise. I have occasional sensory overload, which makes my brain spark and my muscles flinch when I feel nervous. Silence, I can deal with, but noise is the one that is a problem for me. Noise can be too much, especially when babies and toddlers scream loudly. The practice has a small play area where

---

BOX 17.2 ■ Autism Explanation

Autism: Is not an illness or a disease. This is something people are born with and people with autism may find it difficult to communicate, interact, understand how others feel or think, take longer to understand information given to them, they may get anxious or overwhelmed around loud noises, bright lights, and social settings (NHS, 2019b).

children can have books to read and a playhouse to use, which takes up the most space, so they are lucky as they are kept entertained. The loud 'ding dong' noise that accompanies the next patient's appointment happens suddenly and can be disturbing to me. Not all the time though since I stay on high alert for when it is my turn whilst watching the adverts.

Both are accommodated on a TV screen, which shows an endless repetition of PowerPoint presentations on *how smoking is bad for you, why people should eat healthy, and information* on various groups to join like art clubs or other classes. But when I hear the 'ding dong', a name appears on the screen, showing a person's title, full name and what room they need to go to for their appointment. If you ask me, it's a little Too Much Information (TMI) but it's better than someone calling out your name and losing their voice, right?

What makes it worse is the fact that everything constantly changes at my GP practice.

Since I can remember, my usual GP would only work occasional days; she was semi-retired at the time of my visits prior to the coronavirus pandemic but seeing a different GP or Practice Nurse was like a *what should I do or say* situation. Some of the GPs and nurses I met were very kind and most of them understood my needs, which made each appointment positive but the only time I got to see the same GP/nurse was when I started using contraception.

When I got older, my Mum would ask me a question like *is there anything I wanted to say?* during my appointment or *do I have any questions?* Generally, I don't ask questions, but I had more say as time went on. I began to feel comfortable talking about my needs as I reached my late teens, but I still wondered *what will happen next time?* I don't have many skills required for booking appointments because I feel uncomfortable about using a landline phone. I never tried or thought about booking online; I worry that it'll get too complicated. I may consider it one day but, in the meantime, I'm happy for my mum to do it on my behalf.

Hospitals were a different story. I have been to a few and some of them have been positive like having blood tests because of my epilepsy medication and seeing my neurologist on 6 monthly catch-ups. But there are some which have been very negative, and one of the worst I encountered was the one time I had to go into Accident and Emergency (A&E) after a seizure. The treatment I received at my local hospital highlighted a serious lack of training and a poor level of patient care.

My second seizure occurred in 2015, just before Christmas. I was still at drama school at the time, but this was my first full tonic-clonic seizure (Box 17.3).

The first one had happened 7 years ago on a trip, when I blacked out on a coach on the way to France. I didn't know how long I was out, but I didn't go back home. When I was in France, a doctor from the group came to examine me in the hotel where I was staying. He told me that I must have been tired since I left early every morning to go to the airport. So, I just brushed it off and never considered epilepsy.

> ## BOX 17.3 ■ Epilepsy Terms
>
> Tonic = stiffening and clonic = rhythmical jerking.
> During this seizure all the persons muscles will stiffen, and the person will lose consciousness and fall to the floor. The person may bite the inside of their mouth and tongue during this as a result, causing harm. A person may lose the control of their bowel or bladder during this too. Seizure generally last for up to 3 minutes long. If they last longer than 5 minutes or a person has more than three in a row continuously – you call 999 as they made need treatment. When a person comes round from the seizure, they may be very tired, irritable, and confused. It is important to support and reassure the person as much as you can (Epilepsy Foundation, 2017).

The same event happened in 2015 when I woke up early for a class session at drama school. I was talking to my mum at the breakfast table when without any warning, I blacked out. When I came too, the first thing I saw was one of my dogs laying down on the floor beside me. She was close to my body, and I was grateful for her company. I also felt pain on one side of my tongue and inside my cheek. I felt dizzy but the noise was unbearable when I heard her barking. The next thing I remember was two paramedics checking me before carrying me off to the ambulance. I couldn't stand properly, so I had to be supported by the two men carrying me underneath my arms. I was laid down in the ambulance and rushed off to hospital. I couldn't take in my surroundings in the ambulance, but I remember seeing the sun rising (which hurt my eyes) and my mum sitting beside me.

When we arrived, I was put on the stretcher and left to wait inside the A&E room. I saw the bright hospital lights shining above me which really hurt my eyes and overwhelmed my senses. I also remember hearing screaming, which was painful. It turned out that someone who was in the same room as me had been involved in a serious car accident and there were parts of his body that were shattered with the damage that was caused in the crash, including a shard of glass that got stuck in his head. I waited for a long time before I was moved to a bed in a day ward where I stayed for 9 hours. I was on a drip, and it was difficult to move my arm. We waited for hours without seeing anyone and a few times, I asked someone to switch the lights off. One doctor said no but my parents did turn them off, only to have them turned on back again by a nurse a few seconds later. I shut my eyes for most of the visit. I was given no food to eat because of my dietary requirements, so my dad had to go to the hospital shop to find something for me to eat. No luck, everything contained gluten or lactose. There was lots of chocolate but no fruit and the only drinks apart from water were energy drinks. So, lunch was a packet of crisps and a bottle of water.

However, all was not lost as I was referred to a neurologist and I went on a diagnosis process for my epilepsy; I was diagnosed with epilepsy 9 months later.

BOX 17.4 ▪ Quote from Claire Carmichael

Claire: 'At my surgery patients can book double appointments and request a quieter time of the day, so that they aren't waiting in a loud waiting area. This really helps patients. Please, take the time out to help your patients feel comfortable during their appointments. It's shocking Sez has had such poor care!'

With all my experiences at my GP and that experience at the hospital, I realised that there has been a lack of training to support patients with various conditions like autism, learning disabilities and epilepsy. Readers will find it shocking but it's something that doesn't happen to just one person; it's something that occurs every day for many individuals, their families, and carers. However, like I said before, every GP clinic and hospital is different and I'm sure there are nice ones out there (Box 17.4).

Staff training frustrates me, especially where it's little or none. I am sure there are reasons for this but for patients with these difficulties, it is a very important issue that needs to be addressed. No practice or hospital should become a stressful environment for staff or patients. I mean, it wasn't the original intention, right?

We have been lucky to have the National Health Service for over 70 years. Having free care for all is like winning a jackpot in the lottery unlike the healthcare in America (which I had experienced while I was ill on holiday). It is heart breaking to see and I cannot imagine the frustration for families who cannot afford to pay for medicine, care, or food to eat. Having to pay $300 (roughly £200 in UK money) for a box of pills for food poisoning would be too expensive for a family living on a low wage.

But even though we are lucky, why hasn't training improved for doctors, nurses and even the administrative staff? There should be plans to make reasonable accommodations for patients who aren't comfortable with noises or lights that cause sensory overload or who have specific dietary requirements? A different approach is needed for patients who have communication difficulties or even are non-verbal. As a young adult, I only want to be treated with some respect and compassion. Sometimes language could be modified or simplified so that people with less communication skills can feel included in the process that involves them.

I wish I could have the answers to these issues but really, I think it's doubtful that it will change anytime soon. In an ideal world, just for a start, I would love to see the following:

- Specific training to educate staff on patients with autism
- Patient support training to all hospital staff who deal with patients with additional needs
- Appropriate adjustments centred on the patients' needs

- Sessions where presentations can be given by staff or patients with specific needs and disabilities.

If I was asked to take part in the last point I mentioned, I'd happily agree to do that.

To me the most important thing is that patients with additional needs are not made to feel any more stressed in a medical setting because nobody takes 5 minutes to find out if they are sensitive to lights or noise or crowded spaces or have dietary issues. These are basic things that many people must deal with every hour of every day, and we don't need to add unnecessary anxiety to the list.

Living with invisible disabilities can be challenging; I found that having to deal with the uncertainty of how I will be treated makes me struggle to settle into any medical environment. Having additional needs can create barriers for both patients and staff and therefore training, and the appropriate adjustments are vital.

With the continuation of the coronavirus pandemic, many patients will have had important treatment delayed or cancelled due to the pressure on limited resources. However, as things slowly get back to normal, it would be good to think that some thought and action will be given to the issues that I have raised.

Claire Carmichael: *After hearing Sez's story, what actions will you take to help these patients in future? Please have a look at extra training/research around these topics. It is so important that we help our patients feel welcome, safe and comfortable under our care.*

After hearing Sez's story, what actions will you take to help these patients in future? Please have a look at extra training/research around these topics. It is so important that we help our patients feel welcome, safe and comfortable under our care.

Stephen Wanless (Head of Department for Skills and Simulation and Statutory Mandatory Training For BCU) on Neurodiversity and Studying

Dr Stephen Wanless: 'I'm a nurse by background. I qualified in 1996 with a degree in nursing from the University of Manchester. I have worked in Critical Care Units in Coventry, Birmingham, Leicester and London. I moved down to London to work on a rotational post, and I also completed my MSc in Advanced Medical Practice from Kings College, London. The clinical work enabled me to the clinical requirements that were needed to meet the competencies for my MSc Advanced Medical Practice. I worked through the nursing ranks up to management level. I've been at Birmingham City University (BCU) since I started as a lecturer and then went on to become a senior lecturer; now I am an Associate Professor in Clinical Skills and

Simulation. I completed my PhD in 2015 which has enabled me to not only teach, but work with governments around the world as part of my role at BCU, as well as working with students in the undergraduate curriculum. So, I am a very busy individual.

I was diagnosed as an adult with the neurodiverse condition of autism, which includes sensory processing disorder, dyspraxia and Savant syndrome. Having Savants means I have a photographic memory which is not as great as it sounds.

One of the things that I needed to do was to understand my autism. I went to an all-boys grammar school and in my generation, it was thought being autistic was having a learning disability, which I didn't have. I left school with 14 GCSEs and four A levels. I haven't struggled from an academic perspective, but I do struggle from a social diversity point of view meeting in social circles which means I would much rather stand up in front of 1200 people than speak one to one with an individual. I've talked to several students that are on the spectrum just to show that we *can* do it.'

So, if you are reading this and wondering if you are going to make it if you have some form of neurodiversity – you absolutely CAN! Just make sure you get all the help and support you can from your university and placements along the way.

Every nurse was drawn to nursing because of a desire to care, to serve, or to help.
                                    CHRISTINA FEIST-HEILMEIER, RN

References

Epilepsy Action. (2021). *What is epilepsy?* Retrieved from https://www.epilepsy.org.uk/info/what-is-epilepsy. Accessed 7 June 2021.

Epilepsy Foundation. (2017). *Tonic-clonic seizures.* Retrieved from https://www.epilepsy.com/learn/types-seizures/tonic-clonic-seizures. Accessed 7 June 2021.

NHS. (2019b). *What is autism?* Retrieved from https://www.nhs.uk/conditions/autism/what-is-autism/. Accessed 7 June 2021.

CHAPTER 18

Imposter Syndrome

Imposter syndrome, I am pretty sure, most people get this, but what is imposter syndrome? To put it in the simplest of words I can think of: it is when someone feels like a phony/fraud of some sort or like you don't deserve the achievements you are getting. It was a term that was first used by a psychologist Suzanne Imes and Pauline Rose Clance in the 1970s.

Furthermore, a research study by Bravata et al. (2019) showed that there is a clear link between imposter syndrome and job performance amongst not only working professionals but students as well. However, not much has been published on how to manage this? Imposter syndrome always hit me during my placements for some reason. I always thought 'someone is going to catch me out and I won't know something', but then I realised, no one knows it all. Some of my mentors would say 'I qualified years ago, and you might have more up-to-date information than me' in a worried tone of voice. It appeared they may have had some form of imposter syndrome themselves at the time. Like I said, I think we all get it at some point in life. I get it now at work; I will dread it when a patient asks me something I don't know because I worry they will think I am incompetent at my job. However, I always say to my patients when this happens, 'there's so much to know and I can't physically know it all' which helps me feel a lot better.

Imposter syndrome is feelings of self-doubt and being incompetent or fraud regardless of education level or amount of experience. Anyone can get this at any level of nursing, from healthcare assistant to chief executive. For me, I think mine stems from not achieving the grades I wanted in my General Certificate of Secondary Education (GSCEs), this really knocked my confidence. So, when I started doing well in my first year at university, I felt like I was a fraud.

What Does Imposter Syndrome Feel Like?

It is like a constant battle with yourself, but also how you feel others perceive you. Even if someone gives you praise for something, you don't believe you deserve it, and you think that others will soon realise the same thing. As a result of thinking like this, you tend to work harder and harder to prove yourself or become 'worthy' of the praise. Over time, this is going to cause a lot more anxiety, guilt and possibly burn out. In a book by Dr Valerie Young (2011) they describe the five different types of imposters.

1. **The perfectionist** – Focuses on getting things right and how to do something. Avoids doing new things to avoid making any mistakes. The perfectionist will want everything in their life to be perfect.
2. **The natural genius** – This one, I feel is the one that fits me. Someone who gains lots of new skills and achievements with little effort. Comes naturally. However, when you have a difficult time or fail something, you feel ashamed, embarrassed and give yourself a hard time.
3. **The rugged individualist (soloist)** – This person wants to do everything on their own, and if they can't do it alone, they feel unworthy and like a failure.
4. **The expert** – Someone who gathers every piece of information about one topic because they believe they should have all the answers. If they don't know the answer to something, then they feel like a failure. (I think this one is also me at times…)
5. **The superhero** – Someone who links their competence to their success in every position they have had (student, HCA, nurse, friend, parent, sibling etc.). To succeed, they will push themselves to the absolute limit to get there. Even when the maximum effort has been reached they will tell themselves, 'I should be able to do more'.

There is no clear reason why imposter syndrome sets in. Vergauwe et al. (2015) have linked this syndrome to different personality traits, such as

- Perfectionist tendencies
- Low self-efficacy or low confidence levels
- Neuroticism behaviours (anxiety, depression)
- Someone who always strives to be the best

Feenstra et al. (2020) suggested that racism and gender bias can also play great factors towards imposter syndrome feelings. They discuss that it is more prevalent in women, people of colour and anyone who is underrepresented in the professional environment. I have to add here, there is a big difference between imposter syndrome and someone else making you feel that your identity makes you unworthy of your role or achievements. If anyone makes you feel like this, please report it. Don't allow anyone to make you feel this way, it's not right, it could be against the law, and this behaviour needs to be stopped.

How to Handle Imposter Syndrome

1. Recognise your feelings – share them with someone you trust. Sharing these can make you feel less overwhelmed. You might even realise you aren't the only one feeling this way.
2. Create connections/networks – Speak with university friends, colleagues, get that support network around you that will help you and each other. I wouldn't have got through university without my friends; they were my rocks.
3. Challenge the doubts you have – Look at them realistically. What evidence is there to say that you are a 'failure'? Ask yourself, do others *really* think of me

like that, or is this just my brain fooling me? If you were going for a promotion, and you are doubting you will get it, ask yourself, 'What skills do I have that meet the job requirements?' If you have already applied, you probably have all the skills they asked for, so remove that self-doubt and give yourself credit.

4. Stop comparing yourself to others – we ALL do this. But this is your journey, not someone else's. You are an amazing, independent and unique person; no one is you, and you are not someone else. Also, remind yourself, it's ok to take longer to learn something than others. That's ok, who said there is a time frame?

The fact is success doesn't mean you have to get everything right all the time. And success looks like something different to everyone! One person's success might be to get out of bed that day, whilst yours may be to get over 70% in an exam.

Success: is the achievement of something that you have been trying to do
COLLINS DICTIONARY (2022)

It very much depends on what your goals, aims or purpose are, because we all have something different we want to achieve. Life would be boring if we all wanted the same things, wouldn't it? Think about what your aim is, what's your goal (don't forget to those SMART goals we discussed if needed) Concentrate on that, and forget what everyone else is doing around you.

Let no one ever come to you without leaving better and happier.
MOTHER TERESA

References

Bravata, D. M., Watts, S. A., Keefer, A. L., Madhusudhan, D. K., Taylor, K. T., Clark, D. M., et al. (2019). Prevalence, predictors and treatment of impostor syndrome: a systematic review. *Journal of General Internal Medicine, 35*, 1252–1275. Retrieved from https://doi.org/10.1007/s11606-019-05364-1.

Collins Dictionary. (2020). *Definition of success.* Retrieved from https://www.collinsdictionary.com/dictionary/english/success. Accessed 14 September 2020.

Feenstra, S., Begeny, C. T., Ryan, M. K., Rink, F. A., Stoker, J. I., & Jordan, J. (2020). Contexualizing the imposter "syndrome." *Frontiers in Psychology.* Retrieved from https://doi.org/10.3389/fpsyg.2020.575024. Accessed 11 July 2021.

Vergauwe, V., Wille, B., Feys, M., Fruyt, F. D., & Anseel, F. (2015). Fear of being exposed: The trait-relatedness of the imposter phenomenon and its relevance in the work context. *Journal of Business and Psychology, 30*, 565–581. Retrieved from 10.1007/s10869-014-9382-5. Accessed 11 July 2021.

Young, V. (2011). *The secret thoughts of successful women: Why capable people suffer from the impostor syndrome and how to thrive in spite of it.* New York: Crown Business.

CHAPTER 19

LGBTQIA in Healthcare

Disclaimer, this section may trigger a response. It discusses the abuse some people go through, and there are a lot of emotions in this section. Mainly because I have seen it first-hand myself and it makes me so upset that anyone could ever treat another human being so badly. This section is aimed to get you thinking about how to treat patients.

Gender reassignment (from one gender to another) and sexual orientation are protected characteristics of the Equality Act (2010). It is a criminal offence to discriminate against these groups of people, so please bear this in mind when treating patients and working with your colleagues. Regardless of your opinions, religion, culture, upbringing or thoughts, you must always treat everyone you meet with respect, dignity and equality. I wanted to create this section to hopefully help you understand a little more about this community and give you some advice and tips on how you can be more supportive.

We all get it wrong sometimes; we may unknowingly say something that isn't the correct terminology for some patients. Mistakes are made, but it's important that we are open, honest and correct them when we realise we have made them. And from my own experience, patients are always understanding when we make mistakes and apologise to them.

In my opinion, there are not enough healthcare services for Lesbian, Gay, Bisexual, Transgender, Queer (or questioning) (LGBTQ+) people in this country. In fact, it's not just my opinion, I'm sure it's a fact! According to the NHS (2020), there are only nine NHS Gender Identity Clinics (GIC) in the UK! Nine. How many transgender patients do you think there are (that we know of)? The government doesn't know exactly how many there are in the UK, because there has never been any real data collection on this until the recent Census (2021) survey. This survey gathers personal information about everyone in the UK to form statistics about who lives in the UK, including (list not limited to) gender, age, country, career and education. The Government Equalities Office (2018) has estimated that there are around 200,000 to 500,000 transgender people in the UK. Imagine that 200,000 to 500,000 people, and only nine clinics to see them. And that's only the people they know about; it's probably far higher than that. And these clinics are spread across the UK, so a lot of people, I imagine, will have to travel to get to one of these clinics after a huge waiting list which is 4 years for your first appointment (GIC, 2022). The Stonewall (2018a) survey showed these worrying statistics:

1. One in eight transgender (trans) people have been physically attacked by a colleague they work with or a customer.
2. 51% of trans people have hidden their identity at work in fear
3. 25% of trans people have been homeless at some point
4. 34% of trans people have been discriminated against because of their gender identity
5. 44% of people avoid certain streets because they didn't feel safe there
6. 25% were discriminated against when searching for a house/place to rent or buy
7. 41% of trans people have said healthcare staff lacked knowledge of trans health needs

And the last statistic found is exactly why I have included this section in my book. More awareness is needed out there for this group of people. These statistics have increased over the last couple of years I'm sure because the amount of social media posts I have been seeing of people being attacked in the streets for who they are, has risen.

So, someone wants to change their gender? What does it really matter to anyone else other than that person? That person isn't going out there committing a crime; they are just trying to become the person they were meant to be in the first place. Think of it another way: you have gained weight, your nose is too big, your breasts are too small, you hate the freckles on your arms, you have wrinkles and grey hair – you hate a lot about your body, but what can you do? Or what would you do? You would try and fix it in some way – you would dye your hair, maybe get Botox, you would change your diet and exercise to lose weight. Or imagine being born with an extra growth that really affected your mental health because you couldn't bear to look at it. You would go to your doctor and try to get surgery to remove this, right? This is all someone who is transgender wants to do – change their body so they are comfortable and happy in the skin they live in and be who they should have been. However, it's not as easy as going to the supermarket for a hair dye or to the GP for a removal. How long do you think the waiting list is for gender reassignment? YEARS, and I don't mean 1 to 2 – I mean years. I know someone who is still on the waiting list 10 years later. The Gender GP (2020) shows some real-life case studies and how long they have waited just for their first initial consultation on the National Health Service (NHS) at a gender identity clinic (GIC). The wait *starts* at 2 years, in which one person had a letter from the clinic after 2 years just to tell them to stop smoking. Way more needs to be done for these people. Forty-eight percent of transgender people in the UK have attempted suicide at some point in their life; this was taken from a sample size of 889 people (Stonewall, n.d.a). How many more has there realistically been? and think about why this is. Is it because of waiting times of surgery? Is it the discrimination, harassment they face? Is it because their families have turned against them? Or could it be a combination of all of the above? Imagine, someone is going through all of this, and now they are suddenly your patient in front of you. You don't know their background, what they have gone through, or how they have been treated previously. But here they are as your patient today, something you do or say, the way you mistreat this patient just might be the final nail to their coffin. This is why it's important to treat every single patient you see with dignity, respect and kindness: you don't know the battles they have gone through.

STORY TIME

When I was 15 to 16 years old, I had a pretty bad relationship, which we won't go into, but for the purpose of this story, my boyfriend at the time was called Rick (name has been changed for confidentiality). Rick thought he was God's gift to women, and he also thought he was a tough guy. No one messed with Rick or his group of friends. Anyway, one night, my best friend at the time, Ed (name also changed for confidentiality), was coming over to my house to stay for the night. Ed was the loveliest, funniest gay guy I knew. In fact, I think he was probably the first gay man I was ever friends with. We used to have such great nights out together, anyway, but Rick didn't like gay people; I don't know why. He thought being friends with them would turn him gay or give him some form of weird unknown disease maybe? Why are people so homophobic? Who knows? I was always brought up to love everyone and be kind to all. I don't care what race, sexuality, gender or ethnicity you are, I will always be kind to you and love you for who you truly are.

So, back to the story, sorry. One night Ed was coming over to my house to stay over. When he arrived at my door, his face was covered in blood. Gosh, just the image of it now makes me shiver and gives me goosebumps – awful! On his way down my road, Rick and his friends had circled Ed in the street and decided to beat him up there and then, for being gay. JUST for being gay, being in love with someone! I was absolutely LIVID! I was so angry; I felt the blood rush to my face. I'm not too sure why, but I grabbed an Allen key and went to run out the front door to hit them with it. Haha, I'm not sure that would have done a lot of good. Luckily, my mum locked the door before I got to the door handle. So, I decided shouting out the window at them and cursing them was more appropriate. Ed didn't call the police; he wanted to just leave it there. Safe to say, me and Rick didn't last.

This was the first time I had ever seen what hate crime does to someone – being beaten up for being who he is? Loving who he loves? Not hurting anyone else at all. It makes me feel sick to my stomach that anyone can do such a thing to another human being.

In the UK, there are around 1.2 million people who are over the age of 16 who are lesbian, gay or bisexual (ONS, 2018). How many of these people do you think have suffered from some form of abuse or hate crime? One in five LGBTQ+ people has been recipient of hate crime in the last 12 months.

Shockingly, 13% of LGBTQ+ people have had some form of unequal treatment in healthcare from staff, and 23% have witnessed discrimination in healthcare due to being LGBTQ+ (Stonewall, 2018b). This shouldn't even reach a statistic. We shouldn't be allowing this to happen in healthcare. Another reason why this section needed to be here. No matter where someone comes from, who they are or who they want to love, you should be treating everyone as an equal human being. Because that is what they are. I must remind you, discrimination against anyone who is LGBTQ+ is a crime, it is illegal, and the person can press charges, and you will be struck off the NMC register before you have even qualified. Not that any of you reading this would do such a thing (I hope). But if you witness anything like this, please say something, report it and do not just walk away and ignore it. Educate other healthcare professionals about this and make other people more aware; the more we can do for this group of people, the better. And this goes for other groups of people who are often discriminated against – people of colour, people with disabilities, people from certain countries etcetera. Now imagine being someone with one of these AND were LGBTQ+. How do you think they are treated out there? I dread to think.

I was recently scrolling through TikTok (in case you don't know what this is, it's a social media platform purely for videos), there was a teacher on there who is a lesbian and talking about a child at school asking if she had a boyfriend? She said 'No, I have a girlfriend' to which the boy replied 'I didn't know you could have a girlfriend; can boys have boyfriends?' and she replies, 'yes' and then the little boy says, 'that's great, that means there are more people in love then!'. It was such a gorgeous video. However, with everything, there is always one person who has to bring it down. There was a reply in the comments to this video that said, 'it's not your place to discuss this at school!' How would you approach this? If someone asked you if you were married, had a boyfriend etc., would you tell a patient? If you identified as LGBTQ+, would you disclose this to your patients? It's really upsetting that people should have to hide and lie about who they are and who they love.

And I can't lie, I have done it myself; I have lied about having a partner because it was easier than having that conversation and having someone judge me for my relationships. Oh, my sexuality – pansexual. Pansexual means; I fall in love with the person for them regardless of what's under their clothes/their gender. I was always confused about my own sexuality growing up, to be honest. Nothing ever seemed right to me; I didn't feel like I fit into any particular box; sometimes I even referred to myself as a 'free spirit'. But I discovered pansexuality was a thing, and it made perfect sense to me. It does not matter what gender, what organs someone has in their body. I love all the little things that make a person – their mannerisms, the way they smile and talk, the way they see the world, how kind someone is etc. But growing up, it was just easier to say 'I'm straight' or 'I'm a lesbian'– it was always one or the other. One day we may live in a world that is open and free, wouldn't that be lovely? Where no one judged anyone else, everyone

TABLE 19.1 ■ Terminology

Terminology	Meaning
Lesbian	Women who are attracted to women
Gay	Men who are attracted to men
Bisexual/Bi	People who are attracted to more than one gender
Pansexual	People who are attracted to the person and not their gender or sex
Transgender/Trans	A person whose gender identity doesn't match the sex which they were assigned to at birth
Transgender man	Assigned as female at birth but is now a man (or lives as a man)
Transgender woman	Assigned as male at birth but is now a woman (or lives as a woman)
Transitioning	Steps a person takes to align their physical body with their gender identity, which may or may not involve hormone therapy/surgery. But not all trans people will do this. Everyone has their own journey.
Cisgender/CIS	A person whose gender identity matches the sex they were assigned to at birth
Asexual	Someone who doesn't feel romantic attractions to others.
Non-binary	People who don't feel like a man or a woman. Not associated to any gender.
Gender dysphoria	A clinical term for discomfort experienced due to a person's gender identity not matching the sex they were assigned at birth
Pronoun (He/she/they/them/Ze/Zir/their name etc.)	Words to use to refer to people's gender in conversation which varies depending on their gender identity. For example, She/Her, He/Him, They/Them

Stonewall. (2018b). *LGBTQ+ facts and figures*. Retrieved from https://www.stonewall.org.uk/cy/node/24594. Accessed 11 July 2021.

just accepted anyone as they are, and everyone was just kinder, and no one had to 'come out'. See Table 19.1 for some of the LGBTQ+ terminologies used.

Transgender people can also identify as lesbian, gay, bisexual, pansexual, etc. I follow a few people on my social media who are transgender, taken steps such as hormones and surgical procedures to change their body, but are non-binary. So, they do not feel any gender and go by the pronouns they/them. People can struggle with neutral pronouns such as 'they/them', I think this is because, throughout society and upbringing in the world, it's been created and changed through time to show women should look a certain way: 'pink colours, breasts, long hair, make-up, heels, dolls as toys when a child' and boys 'short hair, penis, playing with cars as a child, the colour blue, facial hair etc.' We associate these physical attributes with a certain gender as a result. This means people's brains have these learnt behaviours growing up of 'he/she' rather than 'they/them' when associating the way someone physically appears to us what they are. Just because someone does not have a womb, does not mean they cannot be female, and just because someone doesn't have a penis, does not mean they cannot be male. My mother, for example, had a total hysterectomy and barely any breasts; would this make her a man all of a sudden? No. She was still a woman, because being a woman, man or person is more than biology and appearance. And this isn't a new thing – transgender people have been around for centuries and accepted. It was only in more recent years things changed, laws came in, and hate crimes began. I haven't found the exact reason as to why these suddenly came in; but it is well documented in history that dated back to 200 BC that trans people were accepted and around (Human Rights Campaign, n.d.).

If you do not know what gender someone is, just apologise and ask what their pronouns are. They would rather you do this than just assume and get it wrong. Calling someone by their correct pronoun or gender or preferred name can really make a huge difference to them. And this was one of the first things I was taught as a student nurse: you introduce yourself and then ask the patient their preferred name. We should be using and doing this for every single patient we meet.

STORY TIME

As a GP nurse, I had a young transgender male patient, under 15 years old, with his mum. On the computer system, it said the old name that they were assigned to at birth (their deadname), but in brackets it said 'preferred name' – let's say John to maintain confidentiality. I called the patient by his preferred name, John, into my room with his mother. The mother came into the room, and the first thing she did was a give me huge smile and thank me. Her words were, '*Thank you so much for calling my son his real name. It means so much to us!*'. It makes me well up, teary-eyed now, thinking back to that moment, how grateful they were – that one simple thing made such a big difference to someone's life. It was so wonderful to see how supportive his parents were of his transition too, as I had seen many stories on social media of how awful it can be for some.

One in four trans people has experienced homelessness in their lives, and 1 in 10 trans people aren't supported by their families during their transition (Stonewall, 2018b). And these statistics were taken from a survey in 2018, I suspect, these numbers are far greater now in 2022, but it also depends on who reports them too. Not everyone will have reported this, so the numbers may be even higher than this. In fact, 88% out of 108,001 transgender and non-binary people did not report it according to a recent survey (Stop the Hate, 2021). I wonder if this is what is happening in healthcare too. Are people too afraid to report bad care? Fear of further discrimination maybe? Is this the reason why there has been a lack of education about transgender healthcare in schools, universities and healthcare settings? I can only assume. However, what is clear is that more needs to be done out there.

All of which is so upsetting to think about; no one should be discriminated against, especially by their own family, friends and people they trust, such as healthcare professionals.

I'm going to digress for a small moment, to try and explain the science (or what I think the real science is behind someone being born into the wrong body) because as healthcare professionals we always must go by evidence-based research, and let's face it, there's not enough out there for some things we do. But there is for this, I just don't think anyone has picked up on it yet. Let's go back to the basics: I'm going to ask you a question, and before you read on, I want you to put this chapter down and do some research or thinking or reflecting if that's ok? My question to you is:

'Why Are Men Born with Nipples?'

Because biologically, nipples are created for breastfeeding babies, and biological men can't physically give birth, so why are they there? Some of you may know the answer to this, which is great! But for those who don't know why, here it is.

During pregnancy, when in the womb, the embryo has no known gender when the nipples are created. So, everyone in life, regardless of their gender, starts off as gender neutral (or female, depending on which way you want to view that) and with nipples as a result (LiveScience, 2017). The human is not assigned any gender until weeks later in the pregnancy. My theory is, that something has happened along the way during this phase in pregnancy and the person is born into the wrong body at birth as a result. A mismatch between the body and brain in which some research conducted by Boucher and Chinnah (2020) investigated the anatomy and physiology between the brain and body between cis-gender males and cis-gender females and compared this to transgender people. It was noticed that there is a significant difference between the male and female brains. It was discovered that, in transgender people, their brain anatomy matched that of a cis gender person. So, for example, a transgender man has the brain structure of a cis-gender man; however, their body matches that of a biological female. In conclusion, this research paper found there was a huge difference between the sex (the body's anatomical features) of someone compared to the gender (identity of a person) of them. This just goes to show, this is not a choice for people, people were born this way and I hope this helps understand the scientific evidence behind this, and to show that this isn't just an overnight decision for people, it's very real and very serious.

I had no idea about the issues within transgender healthcare in our NHS. It is only because I started my GP nurse role, I had a transgender patient and I wanted to look more into this and the type of hormones etc that I would be giving to my patients. However, when asking and searching, I could not find any training on this. There is no transgender healthcare training out there at all, in fact. There's a huge gap in many areas of healthcare for our transgender patients. And the more I looked into it, the more I witnessed inequality and discrimination happening.

It was very eye opening and shocking to see the maltreatment and discrimination against this community. I now do everything I can to raise awareness and hopefully create change for the future of our transgender patients and colleagues. I researched every moment I could in my spare time over the next 18+ months (and am still researching today), to gain more insight. I took to the internet to go over guidelines, research papers, articles and talked to many trans people about their experiences out there in healthcare. Alongside this, I visited the London Transgender Clinic for the day to shadow their nurses, and it was amazing to see the work they do! I cannot praise the clinic enough for what they do there. It is a private clinic, but they have so much passion for what they do. It's amazing to see I was actually offered a job there; however, I couldn't commute to London, sadly. From all of this, I started to create webinars to educate students and primary care staff out there on transgender topics. These became so popular, and I realised this was a far greater need than I realised. I had quite a few inboxes asking for more to be put on, and companies wanted me to deliver these to their staff. This was fantastic to see! I then had them implemented across Birmingham primary care teams to educate all staff out there. Slowly, things were progressing, and I needed to create some form of professional organisation with it to gain more credibility. So, I went off and created my own website and social media platforms. I have been joining forces with charities as well to help, such as the Eve Appeal (a charity for gynaecological cancers). It's amazing how one small idea can create such a ripple effect and make a difference out there. The feedback from the webinars has been amazing. The reason I wanted to share this here is because I wanted you to know that just because something isn't already out there doesn't mean that you can't create it. If you are so passionate about something, go for it! Do the research, spend your time creating what you think will make a difference out there and achieve it. I wasn't knowledgeable at all in this field, and suddenly with research, visits and gaining a way better understanding of guidelines, I became an almost semi-pro in this field. And my final say on this topic: please, do some research on this area and do all you can to give your transgender patients the respect, dignity and equality they deserve, just as anyone else you care for. No one should be treated differently just because of their gender.

Case Study by George Blake – A Proud Transgender Man and Residential Support Worker

Hello everyone, I'm George Blake and this is my journey to becoming me.

I write this as a proud trans man, but that wasn't always the case, well to be honest, it wasn't the case at all. Rewind to 1989, when I was born, I had a good upbringing, but I knew early on in my life that something was different about me. Growing up, I was always a tomboy and wanted to play with boys and playing classic childhood games like 'mummies and daddies' I never wanted to be mum; I wanted to be dad. At the time, I never thought anything of it, but looking back, all the signs were there. As you can imagine when puberty hit, it was a whirl-wind of emotions. Having parts developing that you didn't want and knew you shouldn't have and seeing how your friends are getting boyfriends and knowing you wanted that, but you wanted to be the boyfriend. All I can say is that as a teenager with hormones running wild, it was a very confusing time. I had a lot to deal with when it came to school, as I got bullied for the majority of my life for having long, curly hair, being tall with broad shoulders, and being mixed race, so for me even thinking about being a boy was not an option. I remember watching a TV show called 'The L Word' (an LGBTQ+-based drama), and there was a character in there called Max, he came into the show as a woman and then tran-sitioned to male. This was the first time I had seen anything like this on TV or any sort of representation of transgender people for that matter, unfortunately for me the show made this character come across as very aggressive and controlling, which as you can imagine scared me half to death. At that point I put my gender identity to the back of my head as best as I could and tried getting on with my life. I came out as a lesbian and tried to live my life the best way I could and try and forget about how I really felt. Throughout my life I have never been settled, I've had to deal with racism and homophobic things thrown my way, and although they were terrible things I've had to deal with, I always thought it could be a lot worse because being lesbian seemed to be more accepted than being transgender.

Fast forward to when I turned 30, where I had gotten to a point where I couldn't keep living like this anymore, like I said previously I was very unsettled and had a failed marriage, and nothing I did ever seemed to make me happy. I remember I was on holiday with my friend and we had an open and honest dis-cussion, and she turned to me and said that her mum had said, and I quote, 'even though George smiles and seems happy, I can't help but think George would be happier if "she" was a man' and that's when I looked at my friend, cried and said her mum had got it spot on.

Coming to terms with who you truly are is one of the most, scariest, yet, amazing things I have ever experienced. I came home and had the conversation with my family, and they have been so supportive, and even though I was scared, I also felt like a weight had been lifted off my shoulders. I knew I wanted to go on hormones and have surgeries to make my body match the way I felt on the inside, so I knew I would have to take the steps with and have a discussion with my doctor to get me referred to a GIC. As I sat in the doctor's office and told her how I was feeling (and broke down in tears yet again), she reassured me and was very comforting and helpful. She admitted she had never dealt with a trans person before, but she reassured me she was going to do research and look into how they could refer me to a GIC. Within a couple of weeks, she got back to me and got my referral done. I then had my blood, weight, height and body mass index (BMI) done and sent it all off, and she assured me that I should hear from them within 6 months. As you can imagine I left the Dr's feeling positive, thinking my time is nearly here and that I can start living my life the way I was meant to. Fast forward nearly a year later, and I still hadn't heard anything from the GIC clinic; my mental health had gone downhill, and I hated looking at myself in the mirror. I decided to get in touch with the GIC directly, so I gave them a call to see what was happening and if they were any closer to seeing me. When I got through to them, they informed me that the waiting list was really long and that they were seeing patients who have been on the list for 2 years ago, so they couldn't actually give me a time scale at all. I came off the phone and sobbed my heart out, knowing that I couldn't wait that long. I had wasted 30 years of my life in the wrong body, and I had to do something. I started doing research online regarding private care but saw that it could be quite expensive depending on who you go with. I came across Gender GP (a private transgender healthcare service) and if I'm honest, I can't fault them at all, everything is done online and through video calls, so it takes the anxiety out of travelling anywhere. In the middle of all this, I had moved county and lived in a flat on my own and then COVID-19 hit. I was lucky enough to work throughout the pandemic, so I saved and got money together to start my hormones. My GP was happy to do shared care with the private service and had no issues with prescribing my hormones and doing my blood every 3 months. I started my Testogel (testosterone gel that's applied to the skin) in August 2020 and then switched to Sustannon injections (testosterone by intramuscular injection) in January 2021. I have been on hormones now for nearly 2 years, and I can honestly say I have never felt this happy, but I know I'm fortunate that I was able to go private for my hormones and that my GP agreed to shared care, as I know this isn't always the case. There are so many people that turn to the dark market (online/unknown people to get their hormones-a danergous way to do this). because they can't wait for NHS times; they would rather risk putting something in their body not fully knowing what is in it than not do anything and just wait. We go abroad to different countries to get the surgery done because it is cheaper than getting it done here in the UK. We take that risk because to us it is worth it. Just to give you an insight, I recently went to Poland to have my top surgery done (double mastectomy), and it cost £3100. However, to have that same procedure done here in the UK costs between £6000 and £7000 on average (Gender Kit, 2020), and I have heard of extreme prices of up to £10,000. For us as transgender people, we take that risk whether it will put us in harm's way, we do what we need to do to survive. Because for some of us, this is life or death.

We have to jump through so many hoops to prove who we are and to be seen for who we are; so please if you do come into contact with someone who is transgender, please just respect them. It takes a lot of courage to take those steps to go to the doctors to start the ball rolling for hormones. You are professionals

TABLE 19.2 ■ **Best Practice**

The Do's	The Don'ts
• Be respectful	• Ask someone what genitals they have
• Maintain dignity	• Ask someone to see what they
• Keep a non-judgemental approach	looked like before
• Use peoples preferred pronouns	• Ask someone what their birth name
• Listen to people	was (dead name)
• Don't put anyone down	• Don't act shocked
• If you make a mistake – apologies	• Don't make comments such as 'oh
• Do some research	wow you'd never tell!'
• If you don't know ask	

and are meant to provide us with a safe space, so please remember and respect that because you could be the first person they have openly told, and the impression you give them will stay with them (Table 19.2).

I shall leave you with some quotes from the transgender community that I found inspiring:

> *It's revolutionary for any trans person to be seen and visible in a world that tells us we should not exist.*
>
> LAVERNE COX

> *I would like them to understand that we are people. We're human beings, and this is a human life. This is reality for us, and all we ask for is acceptance and validation for what we say that we are. It's basic human right.*
>
> ANDREJA PEJIC

> *Nature made a mistake, which I have corrected.*
>
> CHRISTINE JORGENSEN

Further Reading

GIC, NHS (2022). Waiting Times. NHS GIC. https://gic.nhs.uk/appointments/waiting-times/. (Accessed 03 February 2023). In this issue.

References

Boucher, F. J. O., & Chinnah, T. I. (2020). Gender dysphoria: A review investigating the relationship between genetic influences and brain development. *Adolescent Health Medicine and Therapeutics, 11*, 89–99. Retrieved from https://www.ncbi.nlm.nih.gov/pmc/articles/PMC7415463/. Accessed 2 November 2021.

Census. (2021). *Census 2021.* Retrieved from https://census.gov.uk. Accessed 29 May 2022.

Equality Act. (2010). *Protected characteristic*. Retrieved from https://www.equalityhumanrights.com/en/equality-act/protected-characteristics. Accessed 26 May 2022.

Gender GP. (2020). *The waiting list for NHS gender identity clinics: Patient's experiences*. Retrieved from https://www.gendergp.com/the-waiting-list-for-nhs-gender-identity-clinic-gic-patients-experiences/. Accessed 11 July 2021.

Gender Kit. (2020). *Double incision mastectomy*. Retrieved from https://genderkit.org.uk/article/double-incision-mastectomy/. Accessed 24 May 2022.

Government Equalities Office. (2018). *Trans people in the UK*. Retrieved from https://assets.publishing.service.gov.uk/government/uploads/system/uploads/attachment_data/file/721642/GEO-LGBT-factsheet.pdf. Accessed 11 July 2021.

Human Rights Campaign. (n.d.). *Seven things about transgender people you didn't know*. Retrieved from https://www.hrc.org/resources/seven-things-about-transgender-people-that-you-didnt-know. Accessed 29 May 2022.

LiveScience. (2017). *Why do men have nipples?* Retrieved from https://www.livescience.com/32467-why-do-men-have-nipples.html. Accessed 2 November 2021.

NHS. (2020). *How to find a gender dysphoria clinic*. Retrieved from https://www.nhs.uk/live-well/healthy-body/how-to-find-an-nhs-gender-identity-clinic/. Accessed 11 July 2021.

ONS. (2018). *Sexual orientation, UK:2018*. Retrieved from https://www.ons.gov.uk/peoplepopulationandcommunity/culturalidentity/sexuality/bulletins/sexualidentityuk/2018. Accessed 11 July 2021.

Stonewall. (n.d.a). *Trans key stats*. Retrieved from https://www.stonewall.org.uk/sites/default/files/trans_stats.pdf. Accessed 11 July 2021.

Stonewall. (2018a). *LGBT in Britain – trans report*. Retrieved from https://www.stonewall.org.uk/lgbt-britain-trans-report. Accessed 11 July 2021.

Stonewall. (2018b). *LGT facts and figures*. Retrieved from https://www.stonewall.org.uk/cy/node/24594. Accessed 11 July 2021.

Stop the Hate. (2021). *Transgender hate*. Retrieved from https://www.stophateuk.org/about-hate-crime/transgender-hate/. Accessed 29 May 2022.

CHAPTER 20

Social Media in Nursing

When I started university, we were all warned about social media use. Don't do this, and don't do that, or the Nursing and Midwifery Council (NMC) will have you up in court and throw you off the course. No one told us about the benefits of social media, how to network effectively and how to use it to your advantage. Social media can be such a powerful tool if you just try, and that's why this section is here for you! I discovered the power of Twitter in my second year, and I want to share what happened and also give you some tips and advice to make the most of social media for your future nursing career.

The good news is my university used Twitter quite a lot and promoted it halfway through our first year. During our 'staying successful' event, they had Twitter up on their white screen, showing all their tweets and what people had been tweeting throughout the day. They encouraged everyone to tweet and share posts on the screen which encouraged everyone to join in on the day. It was at this moment, I cleared my Twitter and started to shape it into my nursing social media tool. How did I start this? Here are the first three things I did:

1. I went through all my old posts (there weren't many, as I didn't ever use Twitter) and deleted anything that could be seen as inappropriate.
2. I went through my 'following' list and removed anyone negative or controversial (this isn't needed, but I wanted to avoid accidentally 'liking' a post I shouldn't have).
3. I removed any images that could be seen as 'unprofessional'.

These steps aren't *necessary*, but I wanted to clear my account ready for a fresh new start with my nursing profile – you could just set up a new account. I was going to do this, but I already had a couple of followers (probably around 40?) and didn't want to lose them haha.

I started using social media a lot more towards the end of my first year of the nursing degree. I wanted to start using YouTube and a blog site as a platform to help other student nurses out there and hopefully encourage more people into nursing by showing the positive sides of nursing. Fortunately, it has worked well for me so far! And some of you reading this may have come from my social media channels - thank you for all of your support. I appreciate all of you.

Some things I always keep in mind when I post anything on social media are:

1. Why am I posting this/What is my aim?
2. Is this going to offend anyone? Or can it be seen in a negative light?

3. Am I using 'friendly' language for all? – This is something I recently discovered actually! I had done a vlog on cervical screening and used some language that was not helpful to someone who was a sexual assault survivor. I had no idea what I had done, so I set up a meeting with this person to see how I can improve and share awareness on this. This is one of my biggest tips here: learn from your mistakes and improve – don't get defensive.

4. Don't post something for the 'follows' or the 'likes' – post what you're passionate about and make a real impact.

5. If I'm going to make a statement, can I back it up with real evidence? Because there will always be one healthcare professional who will comment asking to see it.

Story Time

My social media journey. Like I said, I started with Twitter, YouTube and a blog site (I used Word Press as it was free and easy to use at the time). I started sharing my nursing journey, more so during my GP placement and just how amazing it was. The more I blogged, vlogged and tweeted, the more feedback I received from others and how I had helped them out. It took me just over a year to finally get 1000 subscribers on my YouTube channel! If you want to do YouTube, don't expect it to be a quick overnight success (if that's what you are aiming for). It takes a lot of time and dedication to maintain your YouTube channel and gain interest of followers. But if you keep going and spend time with it, you will be amazing! Although some people have been a sudden overnight success out there – huge well done to those people. I personally didn't start any of my social media for followers, likes or comments; I wanted to make a difference out there in the nursing world, and that's why I chose to use every platform available to me to achieve it. My aim was to make a difference or help someone out there and I achieved that ☺

Anyway, back to the story… During my GP placement, I was doing everything I could to get the message out there about how amazing GP nursing was. I had an inbox on Twitter from someone and I am embarrassed to say, I had no idea who this person was (it was a National Health Service (NHS) England lead nurse!) I was asked if I would be interested in doing a talk with this person at a conference! 'WHAATTTTT!?' Wow… of course, in my head I was having a party and thinking, 'Oh my gosh, this is exciting'. Also, terrified me. On the surface and responding, I was trying to be cool as a cucumber haha.

This was an amazing opportunity to be able to stand at a GP nursing conference and talk as a student nurse to a room full of healthcare professionals. A room FULL of healthcare professionals… imposter syndrome hit me, my fear of public speaking hit me, I began to sweat 'but it's ok, I CAN do this' I kept telling myself. And one thing this person said to me, which helped massively on the day, was 'think about it like this, it's not about you now, it's about helping

> **BOX 20.1 ■ NMC Social Media Guidance**
>
> 'Nurses, midwives and nursing associates may put their registration at risk, and students may jeopardise their ability to join our register, if they act in any way that is unprofessional or unlawful on social media including (but not limited to):
>
> ■ sharing confidential information inappropriately
> ■ posting pictures of patients and people receiving care without their consent
> ■ posting inappropriate comments about patients
> ■ bullying, intimidating or exploiting people
> ■ building or pursuing relationships with patients or service users
> ■ stealing personal information or using someone else's identity
> ■ encouraging violence or self-harm and
> ■ inciting hatred or discrimination' (NMC, 2019).

other people and making a difference out there', and they were right. Changing my perspective on it really did help. I was still nervous, but nowhere near as bad as I felt. I had two other amazing people up there with me too, which helped ease it.

The day came, and I was standing, waiting to go on stage for this conference. I had planned it all in my head; I was going to stand on stage, with my speech ready, flashcards in hand in case I got side-tracked (as you can tell, with moments in this book, it happens a lot haha). Anyway, we were miked up and ready to go, and then I saw a sofa… we were to go and sit on the sofa to speak. I hadn't prepared for this, 'no!' I'm a bit odd like that; if something doesn't go as I think it will in my head, it makes me anxious. I don't know why. Not only that, I had bright odd socks on and everyone could see them! But I used that as my ice breaker and made people laugh.

I came off the stage and networked with a few people which was great. I met some wonderful people who I had been speaking to on social media already too! It's so nice to put faces to tweets. I sat in on some workshops that were going on too, which was amazing. And of course, I blogged and tweeted all about it and how fantastic it was! I think I may have been one of the first student nurses to ever stand and speak at an event like this. Following this, I was invited to be part of a new network that had been developed by NHS England – The General Practice Nursing Student and Nurse Network (GPNSNN) as an ambassador. This was a new network set up at the end of 2018 by some fabulous people out there.

Through this network, as ambassadors, we did talks to universities, created our own social media account, shared the amazing stuff going on in GP nursing and dispelled some of the myths out there, such as GP nursing is somewhere to retire to or that you can't go into GP Nursing as a newly qualified nurse (I'm living proof that you can). Spoiler alert: I'm now co-chair of the GPNSNN with other amazing nurses.

The NMC (2019) social media guidance states (Box 20.1)

How to Start Vlogging/Blogging/Using Social Media?

VLOGGING

1. Just get started, pick up your mobile phone, laptop or computer device, and just start.
2. If you want to start vlogging: pick up your camera phone and start. Best tips for this: sit in front of a window during the day, the better the lighting the better the quality of your video. I purely use my iPhone (other makes are available) and iMovie to edit my videos. I don't use a microphone or anything else: nothing fancy and all free.
3. Keep videos short and straight to the point – sometimes I go off-topic! But I try to keep videos shorter, so it doesn't bore people. You can always edit things out.
4. Most of the time, I don't plan my videos. I don't have a script – I just talk and edit the bits I don't want. I feel I show my passion this way. But find the way that works best for you and your style.
5. I use YouTube to vlog, but you can also share on other platforms like Twitter, Instagram, TikTok etc., which are limited to how many minutes you can have, sadly. If you use YouTube, record the video in landscape mode or it will upload in a weird format and not a full screen.
6. Don't think about what others will think of you – if you keep thinking this you will never start. Just record, edit and upload.
7. Ask your viewers what they would like to see from you – I often ask mine to see what sorts of things would be useful to them. This helps structure future videos, too.

BLOGGING

1. If you want to start blogging, have a look at free websites to do this. I have always used WordPress because it is easy to use. Other blogsites are available; work out which one is right for you.
2. Don't compare yourself to others – you are you, and this is your story not anyone else's.
3. Write about anything you're passionate about – A lot of people start off by telling their journey. So, one of my first blogs was about why I came into nursing.
4. You don't need a specific writing style – just write and shine! Like I said, this is your writing and your journey.

TIPS FOR SOCIAL MEDIA USE IN GENERAL

1. Stay professional, don't voice opinions without evidence, don't swear, don't share your bad habits like smoking and drinking. Think about posting as a nurse. Maintain confidentiality too!

2. Don't put others down on social media.
3. A healthy debate is ok, but to get angry at others is not ok. Sometimes social media can get you riled up a little when people are posting things you don't agree with. Drop your shoulders, take a deep breath, and move on. Don't get into an argument because it's really not worth it.
4. BE a supporter! Support, follow, like, comment and share other people's posts and achievements.
5. Don't be afraid to follow and tag the big 'wigs'! They are human after all. I'm following a few people, such as Ruth May, our Chief Nursing Officer, and have tagged her a couple of times in posts I have shared.
6. Don't be afraid to share your own achievements on social media.
7. If you want to find more people to follow, look at other people's 'followers and follows' lists and go follow them.

I hope that gives you a few basics to help you get started – you've got this!

SOME TIPS FOR SOCIAL MEDIA NEGATIVITY

1. Screenshot anything you see for evidence.
2. Block the person so you can't see their posts and they can't harass you.
3. If it's on Twitter specifically, you can mute the tweet/thread so you don't get notifications from it – you can also mute people so they don't come up on your news feed (if only life was this simple haha).
   a. Go to the person's main profile page.
   b. Top right-hand corner there are three dots – click them.
   c. There is the mute/block option.
4. Report this person to their trust and the NMC and whatever social media platform they are using Facebook, Twitter, Instagram etc.
5. Do NOT respond to their posts, stay professional. Gather your evidence and report instead, and let the official governing body police this.
6. Limit social media – don't delete your account (unless you really want to of course)
   a. I have seen people delete their accounts due to people being so cruel to them. Don't allow anyone to make you feel this way! Keep being you, keep being amazing and keep sharing positive posts to drown out the negativity. Don't let them win…
   b. I tend to schedule tweets and take some time out from Twitter. I find this helps me in both ways: helping others with tweets and spreading kindness, but also by taking my own time out to rest and recharge.
   c. Put out a post to say you're taking time out and will be back. People will be so kind and understanding. Social media will always be around, however, your health is more important! So, do what's best for you.

Don't allow anyone to bully or harass another person, or worse, a patient! It takes great courage to be able to speak up, but you will be protecting others as a result. If you don't feel comfortable speaking up, then do it anonymously. Tell management/NMC/anyone you are reporting to that you would like to be kept anonymous, and they should hopefully help you with this.

Story Time

I have suffered from harassment online before; I shall not mention where or when this happened or any names due to confidentiality. This has been the most awful experience I have ever faced, and this was from another healthcare professional. My social media experience has always been so positive until this point, and this scared me. I have never been through anything like this before, but the silver lining is, I can add it to the book, and hopefully others will learn from this, and I can give some advice if this was ever to happen to you.

Let's start from the beginning. If you don't know me, I am the sort of person who loves to spread positivity across social media, as well as raising awareness of different issues. I have always gone above and beyond for everyone around me and putting everyone else first before myself.

On this particular day, I noticed a healthcare professional posting on social media, quite publicly, about another healthcare professional; in fact, there were several posts about different professionals over the months, by the looks of it. Their words were quite nasty, and they had put this other person down, and it just wasn't professional at all. It came across as online bullying, to be honest, and it made me feel very uncomfortable to sit and watch and not help in some way. So, I made the decision to make a comment on the post, and I made one comment about how unprofessional this seemed and tagged the NMC so that they could see what they were doing as well. This person then made a comment and then straight away blocked me, and I blocked them and muted the conversation to avoid any further stress on the matter. After I made that comment, the tables were turned on me. This person decided to write posts about me, accusing me of a few things that I was not and just generally being a very mean person about me. This was not just one or two things; there were between 70 and 100 different posts and comments made about me over the course of about 6 months. Anyone who did not know me personally would have seen that and thought awful things about me. Luckily, most people know me and how I am, and they know I am not the things they are accusing me of.

I refused to respond or rise to this. Instead, I took the professional route and started to gather screenshots of it all and ended up having to report this to the NMC. This person got very defensive once they found out I had complained about them, and this made this person much worse. They took to social media yet again; I was stressed; my heart rate and blood pressure had changed; I started feeling faint at work because of it all; I wasn't sleeping or eating properly. I had to go to my manager and let them know what was going on because it was affecting me so much.

It went quiet for a little while. And then I was informed that this person had found my workplace and had started to call up my workplace to get information about me and find out my manager's details to email them a complaint. This absolutely terrified me, to be honest, because I have no idea how this person had found my workplace. I don't share that information anywhere, and not even my best friend knew which clinic I worked at. So, how did this person get these details? And that was the scary thing, so I had to get the police involved. The police were informed; they took my details, screenshots, a 2-hour statement of everything that had happened and said they would get back to me with the next steps as this was now harassment. I then updated the NMC again with the new information.

Once the police had spoken with this person, they then took to social media AGAIN to harass me, tag me in posts and get their followers to target me next. It was horrific! I just wanted to be left alone, all I had done was try to help someone else and ended up with months' worth of backlash for it. This is not ok from anyone, even worse that it's coming from healthcare professionals. As a result, I have taken a huge step back from my social media. Which is a shame because I have always used social media for the good of nursing. I have made many friends and great networks with my social media, and this has just completely changed everything, sadly. No one speaks about the impact these things have on people. But hopefully, I can give some advice that I have learnt from this.

MY ADVICE TO YOU IF YOU HAVE THIS HAPPEN

1. Block the person.
2. Mute the person's profile and any posts they tag you in if you can.
3. Report the person to social media, NMC and police if needed.
4. Seek advice from your local union.
5. Avoid responding to any posts, as hard as that might be, because you automatically feel like you want to defend yourself. But don't. They will use it against you and make the situation worse.
6. Get support from colleagues, family and friends, and take some time out for yourself.

At the time of writing this, it is still ongoing, and I am awaiting the results from the NMC and the police outcome. I had to change my social media handle and turn private viewing on as a result.

To do what nobody else will do, in a way that nobody else can, in spite of all we go through, is to be a nurse.

RAWSI WILLIAMS, JD, BSN, RN, PHD

Reference

NMC. (2019). *Guidance on using social media responsibly* [pdf]. London, UK: NMC. Retrieved from https://www.nmc.org.uk/globalassets/sitedocuments/nmc-publications/social-media-guidance.pdf. Accessed 21 July 2021.

CHAPTER 21

Money-Saving Tips

*Disclaimer: Everyone is different, and everyone will have a different amount of income depending on their personal circumstances. Please use the student finance calculator to work out how much you will receive roughly. (Just search the internet for 'student finance calculator UK' and it should come up for you.)

Being a student is tough… Like, really tough! No one prepares you for the money side of it, so this is why I wanted to try and include some useful tips and advice to help you get by.

Firstly, as a student, if you are earning less than £12,570 (working part-time) a year, you should not be paying tax (as of May 2021). Make sure you contact the government tax department and tell them you are now a student, and they should put this on your record. If they don't know you're a student, they will continue to tax you as normal (but you can claim this back if you are paying tax as a student currently – get in touch with the tax office.)

The first thing I did before I started was worked out my budget. I sat and wrote down a list of my monthly outgoings: rent, phone bill, travel, food – everything I pay out every month. Luckily, I didn't have much to pay out, but I'm happy to share here just how much I paid out and what I had coming in with student finance and National Health Service (NHS) bursary so you can see how I lived as a student nurse. See (Table 21.1).

As you can see, my personal budget was tight as ever! I can't give an exact amount for what I worked part-time as my shifts were all over the place, and some months I didn't do any and other months I did way more because we had holidays etc. at university (uni), so I worked them. This is one of my tips *if* you can do this. Whenever you have breaks at university for Easter, Christmas etc., use this time to work as much as you can (obviously have some time out for yourself though too! Don't burn yourself out). But this is what I did: I worked every hour I could when on 'holiday' so that the extra money would cover me for the months I could work, like when on my GP placement. I put my pay into my savings for a rainy day then, so I knew I had it if I needed it to pay for food/bills etc.

How to Work Out Your Budget by Week

1. Calculate your incomings
2. Calculate your outgoings

TABLE 21.1 ■ **Outgoing versus Income**

Outgoings Every Month (Jan 2017–Dec 2019)	Income Every Month
Rent: £350	Student finance: £200
Mobile bill: £67	NHS Bursary: £450
Bus pass: £38	**Total incoming: £650**
Food bill: £200	I then worked part time to make extra
Total outgoing: £655	to live

3. Subtract your outgoing from your incoming and then divide this by the number of weeks you have each term. This will give you a weekly figure to go by.
Try and avoid spending over your budgeted amount.
Incomings could be things such as:
1. Bursaries
2. Student finance
3. Work
4. Savings
5. Payments from other people like family allowance
Your outgoings could include:
1. Accommodation (rent/mortgage/student flat)
2. Course books/materials
3. Travel expenses
4. Household bills
5. Extras: social events, gym, hairdresser/barber, books, clothes, hobbies etc.
My next tip is, do a job you love! I was so fortunate because I worked in sexual health, which was a pretty nice job! It wasn't that hectic at the time, and I loved the people I worked with, so it made it so much nicer for me.

Tip for when to work: Sundays are *usually* double pay! Depending on where you work… you can get way more money for working on a Sunday than the rest of the week, which works out nicely for the bank balance.

Please be careful when doing extra shifts because you are legally employed by the university and shouldn't be doing more hours than 48 hours a week as per government guidelines (GOV, 2020). **Do not** cancel placement to work, and **do not** miss university lectures so you can go and work a shift – this can be classed as fraud (if you are funded for the course), and if caught, you will be held accountable for this. So, please be careful in what you're doing out there, I know we need to make money to get by but stay safe.

So, once you have set your in and out goings; you know your budget. Now you can start planning for your month. So, for me, I knew I had around £50 a week for food shopping; luckily, it was just me to cook for! I used to buy huge bags of pasta, egg/rice noodles and rice, so I always had a base to make a meal out of. I stocked my cupboards with herbs and spices in jars, so that I always had some flavour to add, and I always kept some tins and frozen food as well, things such as tinned beans, spaghetti, tomatoes, sweetcorn, tuna. Freezer was bits like frozen veg, pizza, wedges, fish, chicken bits etc. So, I always knew I had some form of a meal ready if I needed it.

To save money I would meal prep as best as I could. I don't personally like eating the same meal over and over again. So, what I did (which I still do at times as well to save money) – I used to make my meal for the evening but make double so that I could put some into a tub and have it for lunch the next day, which worked really well! Simple things like stir-fry or pasta worked well for me. But find what works for you and do that. And if you don't mind having the same meal more than twice a week then you can always make a little extra and freeze it for the week. I personally get very nervous about re-heating meat (which is fine to do). But I would just have vegetable stir-fries or veg pasta for my lunches instead of meat-filled, so simple and easy to cook too! I love anything that all went into one pot haha – saves on washing up.

Next Tips for Money Saving

Get student discounts! Don't be shy, ask at every opportunity when you're shopping, when you're out for food, cinema, anywhere. Sign up for a free student account with places, such as **Student Beans website, UNiDAYS website and Blue Light discounts** (there is a small charge for a blue light card now) too. There is the official NUS student discount card as well which was £24.99 for 3 years (Totum, 2021), which is well worth it if you're using it all the time. However, I found I could use the free sites, so seemed a bit of a waste of money for me.

Shop cheap, go to places like Aldi, Lidl, Asda, Wilkinson's, home bargains, and B&M's (other stores are available). Don't be too proud to shop at cheaper stores – it's smart and saves you so much money! This is how I managed to get all my food shopping for £50 or under every week. This is how I still try and shop too! Why pay more for the same foods and drinks etc., when you can get them so much cheaper?

And always ask yourself, 'Do I really need this?' If the answer is no, then don't buy it.

As a student (even as a mature student) you can get a 16 to 25 railcard which gives you a third off trip on the trains. You will just have to fill out a separate form as a mature student, get the university to stamp it and send it off. But if you are travelling a lot by train, this could be a huge help!

Tips for Uni and Saving Money on Hot Drinks

1. Take a travel mug/flask/water bottle with you to uni to re-fill there
2. Take your own tea bags, coffee, milk and sugar etc. with you

3. Ask the canteen/coffee shop if they will just fill your mug with hot water (which will either be free or a very small fee)
4. Also, take your own lunch and snacks

Tips for Books for Uni

1. Have a look at social media groups and ask if anyone has any spare old books you can have. You can get free books this way – you don't need the most current anatomy and physiology (A&P) books, A & P will never change in the body. Save your money.
2. Have a look at sales pages, charity shops and car boot sales for books too.
3. Ask your local pharmacist for an old British National Formulary (BNF) book and if they have any, they will give it to you for free. When you go in, say you're a new student nurse and would like to ask if they have any old BNF books you can have. This is your nursing 'bible' for medications; however, there is a free app as well as a website.

Days/Trips Out

There are so many free things you can do that don't cost a lot. Walking/hiking (if you enjoy that). Having a movie night around your house and invite friends over (get them to bring their own snacks and drinks.) Picnics in parks, free museums, look for student days out/nights out too. Also, if you have Meerkat Movies – you can get 2 for 1 on cinema and meals out. A big tip I discovered online for Meerkat Movies – if you don't have anything to purchase from them, such as insurance. Just get a very cheap weekend break travel insurance. This is what I did, I paid for travel insurance in the UK for a long weekend for a few pounds and managed to get all the perks of Meerkat Movies (this trick may change as years go by). Look out for free events at your uni/local charities.

Some Extra Bits for Making Money

1. Sell things on social media and on selling pages to make some extra cash
2. Get crafty and sell things on social media
3. Do a car boot sale
4. Some charities will pay for old clothes by the kilo
5. You can get extra money for switching banks – have a look around
6. Get paid to complete online surveys (These are free to join, don't pay!)

I discovered ALL of these tips above as a student nurse (minus the car boot sale), because 1 month I *really* struggled for cash. I had no work for a couple of months, and I was paying out more than what was coming in. I don't have family who could have helped me out, so I had to think of initiative ways to make more money as quick as I could. I created some student nurse placement packs, printed them out, laminated, cut and attached them to a keyring pull chain and sold them on Etsy. It took me the whole weekend of non-stop working to get started. But once I had perfected them, finished them and got them onto Etsy, they sold so well! I was shocked at the feedback I got from these too. So, to the first lot of people who bought these first cards – thank you so much. You kept me alive!

Reminder: if you're doing things like this and earning over the set government amount, you need to start paying taxes. Set up a self-assessment online through the government website to do this as a self-employed person. However, if you are not earning over this threshold, don't worry about it.

Let us never consider ourselves finished, nurses. We must be learning all of our lives.

FLORENCE NIGHTINGALE

References

GOV. (2020). *Maximum weekly working hours.* Retrieved from https://www.gov.uk/ maximum-weekly-working-hours. Accessed 10 August 2021.

Totum. (2021). *Totum.* Retrieved from https://www.totum.com/campaigns/nus-extra-is-totum. Accessed 10 August 2021.

CHAPTER 22

Coping through a Pandemic

In March 2020, the World Health Organization declared a pandemic of COVID-19. I remember over Christmas and New Year, watching the news of a new virus that was sweeping across countries. You could see it coming like a tsunami, but our government didn't seem to be bothered by this and suggested it was 'just the flu'. However, seeing this on the news, I knew this was bigger than what they had thought. I had just qualified, but I had worked in healthcare for several years and knew that this wouldn't be good.

I started my first newly qualified post in February 2020, shortly before the pandemic was declared. I remember hearing the news and wondering what would happen to me as a nurse. Would my role change? Would I be relocated? What was going to happen to my colleagues and patients? To be honest, I became obsessed with COVID-19 at the start. I sat and spent my days researching it, reading the science behind it, reading about the history of pandemics, infection control and any latest news briefs. It's far better to be overprepared than underprepared for these things.

In the beginning, everything was new – a new virus and new ways of working. However, it seemed to me that everyone's infection control training had gone out of the window. It seemed people had forgotten, we have had pandemics, epidemics, vaccines etc. before, that part wasn't new. The only new part about this is the type of virus and the damage it does. Infection control policies and procedures have been around for years, and regardless of what virus is around, we should be following the best available evidence we have. Not only that but contact tracing has also been around for years. I worked in sexual health for almost 6 years and learnt a lot about contact tracing and how it works; we had been doing it for years. Yet enter a new virus, and no one appeared to know what to do. A whole new contact tracing app was created, and a contact tracing team was created to help handle this, which on paper looked fantastic. However, like everything, there were flaws in technology being reliable. Anyway, I digress, back to the pandemic working life. One thing we do as nurses and something we have learnt from day 1 is infection control. There are so many research papers on this and a lot of evidence for it. As nurses, we are taught to find the best available evidence to be able to give the best and safest care possible to our patients. Regardless of what our Prime Minister says, we should be following this. So do your research, know your infection control guidelines, policies and procedures, and what the best practice is. People seemed to forget this during a pandemic, and it doesn't matter what a prime minister says, if it's not safe to do so, you don't do it, and if you can justify your action and show you've followed best practice and evidence, you can't go wrong. For example, at the beginning, we were told we didn't need personal protective equipment (PPE) for this 'flu' virus. I had friends working on wards caring for COVID-positive patients without any PPE who then contracted COVID-19 as a result.

Now evidence shows, masks DO protect you and others from harm, it's the reason theatre staff/surgeons etc. wear masks. It's infection control measures which have been proven to work. Later down the line, masks were suddenly mandatory, and I am not sure why they didn't make them mandatory from the start, to be honest; it could have protected a lot more people from day 1. So, please, if you don't agree with a decision made and you can back it up with evidence, please speak up and protect others. Along with this, it doesn't matter what band of nurse you are – whether you are a healthcare assistant, student nurse or qualified nurse – you have the ability to speak up and make change where you are.

Back to my role, I was working as a GP nurse and as no one knew the true extent of the pandemic, all of our clinics were massively reduced. All patients were triaged and prioritised and we only saw patients we really had to, such as for wound management, urgent electrocardiogram (ECG)/blood, and injections. Even with wounds, I taught my patients how to re-dress them at home, gave them all the dressing sets they needed to do so and education round infection control and aseptic technique. Then patients could re-dress from home, and we would review every couple of weeks or before if they noticed any changes/deterioration. This actually worked really well in the clinic I worked in; patients seemed to feel empowered as a result. Wounds appeared to heal better in some way too. I was learning new ways of working, new ways to empower and protect my patients, it was fantastic. I don't mean to offend anyone by saying this, but patients seem to rely on healthcare staff a lot for things they can do from home. It's really important we empower and reassure our patients to take better care of their health and not for us to take 100% of the responsibility.

I had gone from seeing almost 30 patients a day face to face to about 3 patients a day at the beginning of the pandemic. To be honest, this had some positives, I was able to complete a lot of my training, I completed a lot of e-learning sessions and I did research around the pandemic. The death rates had gone up, and the pandemic seemed to be getting worse. I had thoughts that I may be redeployed to the hospitals or community to care for people with COVID-19 at home. I had visions of caring for people who were dying at home because the hospitals were too overwhelmed to help them. I sat and cried just thinking about it all. I had no idea what was going to happen, but one thing that never crossed my mind was fear. I wasn't afraid; I never once thought about catching it myself or dying from it. My first thought was, 'I need to do what I can to help others'. Because this is why I came into nursing, to help others and I would do anything I could for anyone. I was lucky in a way because I didn't have children or anyone at home who was vulnerable, so I didn't have that worry of 'what if I bring it home and give it to someone?' Whereas I know many people cared for vulnerable family members and had children to think about. I remember seeing a video of a nurse in tears on social media, she had witnessed the COVID-19 deaths, fear in people's eyes and then feared bringing it home to her loved ones. Something I was always taught at Birmingham City University (BCU), you and your family come first. Nursing will always be around, but you and your family may not be, so you must look after yourself before anyone else. We often feel guilty for being sick and off work, or we can't pick up an extra shift when it's short at work. However, we can't think that way; we should always care for ourselves, because if we aren't our best selves, then patient care suffers as a result. So please, take care of yourself and your family, always. Nursing will always be here for you when you're ok again.

When the new vaccine was created for COVID-19, it's safe to say we were all extremely proud to be part of the National Health Service (NHS) rollout. Not only excited, proud and ready for the pandemic to end, but nervous. Many of us, myself included, were worried about the new vaccine and how it has been created so quickly and if it would work at all. I'm not proud to say it, but I refused to have my vaccine until I had gone through every piece of research around it first. I was a new nurse, new to vaccinations and immunisations, and wanted to know more first. Once I had done all of my research, I was happy with everything. Research showed that the vaccine was over 80% effective (UK Health Security Agency, 2021) and worked well for the virus, but not only that, the companies making the vaccines are not new. These companies have been making our vaccines and immunisations, along with other medications, for years and years. It was purely for a new virus that's all. And given how effective all the other vaccines are, I'm happy to say I had mine straight away.

As a GP nurse, I was part of the vaccine rollout, I will never forget the first day I gave my first vaccine. It was such an emotional moment, knowing I was going to be part of helping reduce COVID-19 and be part of history. I remember the patients all being really emotional and happy as well. Mostly, people thanked us and brought cakes and chocolates to thank us; however, it's not us that should be thanked. The scientists who worked 24/7 to get this vaccine right are geniuses. One of the questions with the vaccine was, 'how has it been made so fast?' a question I asked myself too. When making a vaccine, it can take years, but this is because of the legal issues, red tape, and a lot of hoops that need to be jumped before vaccines are rolled out. However, in a pandemic, that red tape is removed. In a normal research study, different groups of participants tend to be part of the study for months, and then it alternates to another different group of participants for another set number of months, and then another group etc. But there was no time to waste on changing groups of people, so instead, groups were run alongside one another to speed up the process given the pandemic. So, this is how they managed to reduce time and create a vaccine which appears to work very well right now. I know there are a lot of conspiracy theories out there on this, but please do your research into it all before believing some of these. It can be quite easy to fall into the trap of a conspiracy theorist and become a non-believer etc. I have doubted things myself as a result of seeing people's stories online along with the government (as in our prime minister's rules) guidelines that keep changing or contradicting one another. But as nurses, we are taught how to research evidence, use this skill, and make an informed choice ourselves. I checked research, found evidence, and followed the science and facts over anything else.

Once lockdown had started to ease, the vaccine rollout of first doses had been done as best as possible, things started to ease a little. I started to see full clinics of patients again, and things appeared slightly more settled, but not over. During the vaccine roll out, all of the practices in our area worked together to deliver this from one big clinic. We all worked evenings and weekends to make this happen. However, people slowly became burnt out and practices decided that for the booster doses, they wouldn't be taking part in delivering them. As staff needed protection and prevention from burning out completely and being off with sickness as a result.

One of my thoughts for the pandemic was that things would change in a positive way; patients would take better care of their health and be more appreciative of healthcare staff, and I honestly thought our government (Boris Johnson, Prime Minister at the time of writing this) would recognise all the hard work we had done throughout and make changes to value the nursing profession. Sadly, this hasn't happened yet, but I am still hopeful. Another thought I had at the beginning of the pandemic was that people would realise the value of life, kindness and generosity. I had an amazing vision that the world was going to change for the better following such a tragedy, but sadly I was wrong here too. Now that the restrictions have been reduced in 2022, people seem to be demanding way more than before. Expecting more from healthcare professionals and demanding services that we just can't provide out there. Waiting lists are far longer than they were before, and people just don't understand the impact of what we have just been through. Nevertheless, I do still lie here in hope of change for a better world, my hope is not gone yet.

Hope is being able to see that there is light despite all of the darkness

DESMOND TUTU

Reference

UK Health Security Agency. (2021). *Monitoring reports of the effectiveness of COVID-19 vaccination*. Retrieved from https://www.gov.uk/guidance/monitoring-reports-of-the-effectiveness-of-covid-19-vaccination. Accessed 4 January 2022.

CHAPTER 23

Ethnic Minority Groups in Healthcare

Firstly, I am a white British woman. I could not write this section without the input from people from different ethnicities. I have had help on this section from friends who do not wish to be named here. You may have heard (or not) of the terms BAME/BME. This stands for 'Black, Asian and Minority Ethnic/Black and Minority Ethnic'. Alongside the term POC, which stands for People of Colour. However, these are terms which can potentially be offensive to people. Recent surveys were completed by the government which showed this.

The language we use and the way we speak to and about people really does matter. Not only that, but it matters within our documentation as healthcare professionals, and we need to be mindful of this. Like many sections within this book, my advice is, always ask the person in front of you. Include them in what you're doing and find the correct language they would like you to use for their ethnicity (Bunglawala, 2019). The Commission on Race and Ethnic Disparities (2021) has given recommendations following research and surveys into the term BAME/POC and they now recommend people use the term 'ethnic minority' instead. This allows for all ethnic groups to be considered.

Inequalities happen within healthcare, and I hate to think that *anyone* would ever be treated any differently purely for their race/ethnicity. It's shocking when you investigate the statistic of inequalities in healthcare in this population group.

What I have found during my research on this, was:

- A BMA (2018) survey found 85% of ethnic minority doctors felt there was a lack of respect for their culture and did not feel included in the workplace.
- Another article by Tonkin (2019) reports that the number of racist attacks increased from 589 to 1448 between 2013 and 2018.
- Another BMA (2017) report showed that ethnic minority students had reported bullying and harassment four times greater than the White ethnicity group. In addition, this report showed inequality in progression into senior roles when comparing ethnic minority groups to people from a White background.

Those are just some of the statistics out there. Overall evidence out there shows harassment, abuse and racism are common themes within healthcare, between staff, colleagues, and patients. It really saddens me that this is happening out there. Some of my best friends are within these groups, and I would hate to think of them ever being targeted purely for their race/ethnicity. It's not right at all! So, please be mindful when you are out there in placement or when working, or just in life in general. Be kind, support everyone you can, and don't be part of the problem. And don't forget, race/ethnicity is a protected characteristic under the Equality Act (2010) and to discriminate against anyone for this, is an offence.

Something I was never taught within university was about diet around Ramadan in cultures. I had to do my own research around this to help gain more knowledge to help my patients. So, I'm hoping I can add some bits here for you that might help you care for your patients during this time too. For those of you that don't know about Ramadan, this is a month where people of faith will fast for the whole month. Fasting happens between sunrise and sunset to allow people to focus on prayer and pure thoughts. The intention of Ramadan is to allow people to understand the suffering of the world (Muslim Hands, 2022). However, during Ramadan, this may affect our patients or colleagues who are diabetic. Diabetes is a problem within the body that alters insulin levels, and your own body attacks itself so that you don't produce enough insulin to allow the uptake of sugar into your cells. Furthermore, some people can manage it through diet and exercise, while others need medications to help them stay healthy (NHS, 2019).

Disclaimer This section is not medical advice; it is taken from relevant resources to help you understand more on the topic. Please do your own research, get advice from medical teams above anything else mentioned in this book.

Diabetes UK (2022) has published a fantastic resource about diabetes and fasting during Ramadan. Mainly due to diabetes, as fasting can alter diabetic levels in the body and cause a deterioration of the person as a result. Firstly, anyone with a health condition who is at risk does not have to adhere to Ramadan. It is accepted that they may be exempt from fasting if this is going to cause medical concern (Abolaban and Al-Moujahed, 2017). However, if people decide to still fast, here is some advice to help monitor this:

- Ensuring patients/colleagues check their blood glucose levels regularly.
- Adjusting medications to accommodate this (a nurse prescriber, doctor or diabetic nurse will do this) – If you need advice, get in contact with your diabetes nurse, who will have all the information to help manage this.
- If blood glucose levels drop, they must break their fast to gain some sugar/starchy foods to help them.
- If levels rise over 16.6 mmol/L, they must breakfast and seek medical advice.
- When breaking fasting, they should eat high-fibre starchy foods, such as oats, wheat, brown rice, lentils and beans, within limits. Alongside, sugar-free drinks to stay hydrated (Diabetes UK, 2022).

To nursing students who are fasting during Ramadan whilst working or studying, here are some tips for you:

- Give your module lead, placement team, supervisor, manager etc. the heads up! Make sure they know you're fasting so that they can adjust for you if needed.
- Start your day earlier if you can so that you can finish earlier.
- Help your colleagues understand what you are doing and why, and educate those around you.
- Take regular breaks and rest to keep you going.
- Take your breaks at different times of the day to accommodate you; employers must justify any requests they deny. If they cannot justify it, this may be discrimination. As long as you are maintaining your work balance, and it doesn't affect the 'business' as such.
- Look at your timetable and see if you can work things around it, if you need to make adjustments to your study, speak to your university to try and accommodate this.

(The Muslim Council of Britain, 2022).

Patel et al. (2020) produced guidelines around risk management of diabetes which are very good and clear to understand. The report shows those at **lower risk are:**

- People with well-controlled diabetes type 2 on a diet or medications and healthy

People at moderate risk were:

- People with moderately controlled diabetes on diet or treatments

People at higher risk were:

- People with diabetes type 1
- People with diabetes type 2 with poor control and poor awareness of their condition
- People who have a history of comorbidities and history of hyperglycaemic episodes within the last 3 months and anyone with a current infection
- Pregnancy

The first-line treatment for patients with diabetes during Ramadan are: (guidelines may change over the years as new evidence emerges, always check the most recent guidelines first):

- Metformin which has a lower risk of hypoglycaemic episodes

Other medications will need to be used with caution, and you should always check with your doctor, nurse or diabetes teams before altering your own treatment or advising others.

Something we were taught in university was pressure area care for people who have dark-pigmented skin. Although it was a very brief session, it was useful and it's something you will 100% need in nursing when doing your pressure area checks on patients. Some research conducted by Gunowa et al. (2018) discovered that people with darker skin tones were more likely to develop pressure damage which was more severe. Additionally, they found that there was a lack of guidance and education around this which may contribute to those results. And this is why I wanted to add this piece here, because I hope it will help you with your assessments of your patients and prevent this from happening.

In a White Caucasian person, the first sign of pressure damage is redness to the skin which does not blanch when pressed. This means that if you were to see a red patch of skin on a patient, you would press your finger against it for a few seconds (not too hard!), and then release your finger; once you remove your finger, if the skin remains red and does not turn white during this time, this is the danger zone. It's the beginning of a pressure area developing. Any redness to skin is a sign of pressure areas; however, if this is non-blanching, it's more dangerous (Shi et al., 2020). However, this is going to be harder to access for people with darker pigmentation of their skin, and other adjustments are needed to assess this thoroughly. It is also important to ask your patient, what is 'normal' for them as they will know their skin better than anyone. Here are some top tips to help you assess this:

- On admission to your services, make sure a thorough skin inspection is documented as soon as possible, this gives you a baseline to assess from.
- After this, examine the skin for any changes in colour or texture of the skin, as darker colours (dark brown/black/grey/maroon/dark purple) or skin texture changes might be a sign of pressure damage.
- Make sure you have good natural lighting to examine the skin.
- Compare areas of the skin to check for differences in their body (Black and Simende, 2020).

Whilst we are on the subject of pressure areas, here is a little bit more about pressure areas, so you gain a better understanding of this:

A pressure ulcer is basically some damage or an injury caused to the skin that stems from pressure being applied to that area and the blood supply has been cut off. For example, if you're lying flat on a hard surface for a long period of time without moving, it's going to block off the blood supply and cause damage and skin breakdown. Because you have that constant pressure on one area over a certain amount of time (NHS, 2020).

Firstly, before we go into the categories of pressure ulcers, I just wanted to say that wherever you're working, there should be a risk assessment in place already where they will risk assessing each patient on admission to see if they're in danger of developing a pressure or if their nutritional status is poor, their fluid balance is poor, or anything like that which could put them at a higher risk of developing pressure ulcers. So, just have a look at your local trust's policies and procedures for how you assess patients and how you do things, and just go from there.

Pressure areas are usually seen in the bonier prominence of the human body so you will have:

- Elbows
- Knees
- Hips
- Heels and ankles

- Spine
- Sacrum
- Shoulder blades
- Ears
- Back of the head
- Toes

(NHS, 2020)

Anywhere that is bony, basically, that hasn't got any fleshy meaty bits that's going to protect it as much as the rest of your body. These are usually due to prolonged pressure on that particular area; this isn't just a short-term thing; this is more of a prolonged pressure over a few hours (Patient Info, 2018).

You might see some red blanching areas which is a sign of the start of the pressure as discussed. This symptom is classed as a category 1 pressure ulcer, and a person should be repositioned more frequently to prevent any further break down of the skin (Office for Health Improvement and Disparities, 2022).

Some extra steps will have to be put in place to protect that and stop the skin from breaking down further, such as using a barrier cream and the skin around it, as long as the skin is intact with no breakages to the skin. If there is some skin loss, and if there is partial skin loss no deeper than the dermic layer of skin, this would be classed as a category 2 ulcer. Sometimes it can look like a small blister or a large blister but there'll be no bruising, no redness, no darkness underneath; it will just be a clear blister which is round (Wound Source, 2022a).

That sort of pressure also should be reported, and it should be documented as well in the patient notes, but the tissue viability nurses don't need to be contacted at this point.

A category 3 pressure ulcer is when there's full-thickness skin loss and there will be some fatty layers exposed, but there's not going to be bone, muscles, tendons or anything like that exposed yet (Wound Source, 2022b). With category 3 you must also report this, and you should also refer to the tissue viability nurses in your local trust.

And that leaves us with a category 4 pressure ulcer. This is a step up again, and you're going to have a full tissue loss; you're going to have muscle exposed, tendon exposed, bone exposed; this might also include what they call undermining or tunnelling (Wound Source, 2022b).

Tunnelling is where the pressure also is quite deep, but there's a little hole where it's tunnelling underneath the skin even deeper, and you can't measure it or know how deep it's going. Because you can't physically see it, that's when you have to get the probe and measure that area to assess how deep this is (Wound Source, 2017). Also depends on where this category 4 is located. If this is on the sacrum area/the buttocks, somewhere that's got a bit of meat to it, then this might be a lot deeper.

There is sometimes confusion between the categories, and you might have a bit of debate with colleagues or nurses about what sort of category this actually is. You might have to get advice from the tissue viability nurse as a result. Some pressure ulcers may be categorised as 'ungradable' which is when you can't see what is underneath them. So, things like, if this was tunnelling, necrotic, black scabbing to the top layer of skin, or so much thick yellow slough to the top of it which is hiding what's underneath. This absolutely must be referred to the tissue viability nurses so that extra measures can be put in place to debride the area. Other causes of pressure area can be healthcare related such as

- Oxygen tuning to face
- Blood saturation probe being left on a finger for too long
- Catheter tubing sitting on skin for too long
- Blood pressure cuffs being left on for too long
- Incontinence pads which also cause moisture lesions (NICE 2015)

And last but not least, the wonderful moisture lesions. So, one of the most common types of moisture lesions I've seen on my patients is because they're incontinent of urine. People can also get them under the breasts, on skin flaps, in groin areas and on the buttocks. You can get these moisture lesions in all sorts of areas, wherever there's moisture, basically. Moisture can be caused by a variety of things such as sweating, urine, faeces, leakage from wounds (Brighton and Sussex University Hospitals NHS Trust 2019)

Whatever pressure area you might suspect, just make sure you are documenting this, informing staff and putting things in place to prevent deterioration and promote blood circulation to the area.

Mish Robinson (Mental Health Practitioner) on Skin Care

Misha was a patient on a particular medication, and the adverse side effects noted on the patient information leaflet were skin rashes/skin discolouration. She raised her concerns with the nurse consultant she was assigned to, but the nurse could not see the skin as any different because she thought it was Misha's normal skin colour. However, Misha knew her skin colour and texture have changed and were different from their normal appearances due to the side effects of her prescribed medications. The nurse consultant dismissed Misha's concerns and did not listen to her. Misha left the appointment feeling unheard and immediately asked to see the original medical consultant who immediately noted the skin rash and discolouration as adverse and stopped the medications. The medical consultant prescribed an alternative which helped her and stopped her side effects. Misha's advice to you is that if you have a patient with a different skin colour, who does not present as White Caucasian, you might have difficulty in assessing their skin. As with any patient you care for you should always:

- Listen to your patient
- Empower your patient
- Be your patient

- Your patient is the expert for their body as they live with it every day
- Include your patient in assessing their skin
- Respect your patient and maintain their dignity

Mish Robinson (Mental Health Practitioner) 18 May 2022 on Leadership

Hello, my name is Mish Robinson. I am a mental health nurse first and foremost; that was my first profession. I love education, hence the reason why I actually did a master's in education. I'm the sort of person who's always studying something, and I've been studying pretty much all my life, I would say. What have I been exposed to? I've been exposed to many different leadership styles in my 30 years of nursing and education. For me, I wasn't really interested in focusing on the climb upward. I'm very much interested in what you can do, and I'm a can-do sort of person. So, I guess I prefer leadership styles which focus on empowering people. So, as mental health nurses, we are about helping people to cope and helping people to move on. So that's where the enabling and empowering attitude comes in. I'm just going to introduce this right now because it's passionate for me. As a woman of colour, I've had decades of being told no or hearing the word troublemaker, and I find that particularly offensive, not least, that was a term given to runaway slaves. These terms are used often without people thinking, which triggers an emotional response.

Claire Carmichael: 'I spoke with Misha about terms and language that might have been used to give an example of what has happened to her, and she said:'

The last time this happened to her was recently (in 2022) at a team launch event at a new job. On arrival at the door, she told them she was there for the event, and the person with the clipboard asked, 'What is your name? I can't see it on the list?' (without knowing her name), to which Misha replied, 'You won't see it on the list if you don't know the name'. The other person stood there chipped in with 'Oh, you're making trouble already'. Misha believes she was judged by the way she looks at this event. I was shocked by hearing this story and just how judgemental people can be. I wonder how a White Caucasian person might be treated in comparison to her at that event? Things like this should not be happening out there, whether at work, on placement, in the community or anywhere in the world. Everyone should be treated equally and with the same respect, regardless of their race or ethnicity. And I hope if you are reading this and you see anything like this happening, to speak up and report it. Let's prevent this from ever happening.

SOME TERMS TO BE MINDFUL OF WHEN SPEAKING TO OTHERS OR THE 'DON'TS'

- Consider how you would want to be treated
- Treat people as individuals and do not judge based on appearance

- Develop self-awareness
- Do not refer to someone as aggressive or intimidating
- Beware of labelling and preconceptions

These are potential trigger words that can really offend someone. It can bring back painful memories of the words associated with the race/ethnicity. Please be mindful and respectful when speaking to others.

That's another thing about leadership; in a way, it has nothing to do with you. It may be about themselves or someone else they've dealt with.

I worked with therapeutic groups; I worked in a day hospital nearly 30 years ago, and this was in mental health. Leadership can work through coaching as well. And I had lots of different therapy training, so I did a couple of years' worth of cognitive behavioural therapy because I found that when you're working in a group, it's about helping people to change unhelpful behaviours and move on to more helpful behaviours. I like thinking about what people *can* do, thinking about the possibilities that I find helps me. So, not focusing on the challenge that much, but focusing on where the change can occur. So being a change agent.

When it comes to leading, it doesn't mean that you have to know everything, but it may be a case of saying, 'OK, I'm not sure about that, but I can come back for you'. I'll find out and come back and tell you, and I think that's better than saying you don't know. Don't present yourself as an expert. So, if you're clear on what you know and don't know, you can lead and demonstrate as an example of how to make a difference in the care you give or with the colleagues with whom you work.

I was a nurse working in higher education. Directing four different professional groups. And I think it's this lack of challenge that we've experienced all these different years that allows microaggressions and covert. Isn't should we say, not just? Racism, sexism, ageism, homophobia, all of that. That's what allows it to continue because no one challenges it. So, you have to learn to challenge. And if you can challenge with kindness, and we all respect ourselves. I wonder if we could do a bit more. And in terms of how we see ourselves and how we behave. How we think and how we feel as informing the way that we behave.

FUN FACT

Only 10.8% of nurses in the UK are men (RCN, 2021).

References

Abolaban, Heba, & Al-Moujahed, Ahmad (2017). Muslim patients in Ramadan: A review for primary care physicians. *Avicenna J Med*, 7(3), 81–87. doi:10.4103/ajm. AJM_76_17. In this issue.

Black, J., & Simende, A. (2020). Ten top tips: Assessing darkly pigmented skin. *Wounds International*, *11*(3), 8–11. Retrieved from https://www.woundsinternational.com/resources/details/ten-top-tips-assessing-darkly-pigmented-skin. Accessed 26 May 2022.

BMA. (2017). *Differential attainment making medical training fair for all.* Retrieved from https://www.bma.org.uk/media/2850/bma-differential-attainment-report-nov-2017.pdf. Accessed 26 May 2022.

BMA. (2018). *Caring, supportive, collaborative: A future vision for the NHS.* Retrieved from https://www.bma.org.uk/advice-and-support/nhs-delivery-and-workforce/the-future/caring-supportive-collaborative-a-future-vision-for-the-nhs. Accessed 26 May 2022.

Brighton and Sussex University Hospitals NHS Trust (2019). Moisture lesionsand incontinence associated dermatitis. https://www.bsuh.nhs.uk/wp-content/uploads/sites/5/2016/09/Moisture-lesions-and-incontinence-associated-dermatitis.pdf. (Accessed 10 February 2023).

Bunglawala, Z. (2019). *Please don't call me BAME or BME.* Retrieved from https://civilservice.blog.gov.uk/2019/07/08/please-dont-call-me-bame-or-bme/. Accessed 26 May 2022.

Commission on Race and Ethnic Disparities. (2021). *Independent report: Summary of recommendations.* Retrieved from https://www.gov.uk/government/publications/the-report-of-the-commission-on-race-and-ethnic-disparities/summary-of-recommendations#recommendation-24-%20%20%20%20%20%20%20%20%20%20%20%20disaggregate-the-term-bame. Accessed 30 May 2022.

Diabetes UK. (2022). *Diabetes and Ramadan.* Retrieved from https://www.diabetes.org.uk/guide-to-diabetes/managing-your-diabetes/ramadan. Accessed 19 May 2022.

Equality Act. (2010). *Equality Act 2010.* Retrieved from https://www.legislation.gov.uk/ukpga/2010/15/contents. Accessed18 June 2021.

Gunowa, N. Q., Hutchinson, M., Brooke, J., & Jackson, D. (2018). Pressure injuries in people with darker skin tones: A literature review. *Journal of Clinical Nursing, 27*(1–18), 3266–3275. https://doi.org/10.1111/jocn.14062.

Muslim Hands. (2022) *What is Ramadan?* Retrieved from https://muslimhands.org.uk/ramadan/what-is-ramadan. Accessed 26 May 2022.

NHS. (2019). *Diabetes.* Retrieved from https://www.nhs.uk/conditions/diabetes/. Accessed 26 May 2022.

NHS. (2020). *Pressure ulcers (pressure sores).* Retrieved from https://www.nhs.uk/conditions/pressure-sores/. Accessed 26 May 2022.

NHS (2020). *Symptoms of pressure ulcers.* Retrieved from https://www.nhsinform.scot/illnesses-and-conditions/skin-hair-and-nails/pressure-ulcers#symptoms-of-pressure-ulcers.

NICE (2015). Pressure Ulcers. https://www.nice.org.uk/guidance/qs89/resources/pressure-ulcers-pdf-2098916972485.

Office for Health Improvement and Disparities, 2022. GuidancePressure ulcers: applying All Our Health. https://www.gov.uk/government/publications/pressure-ulcers-applying-all-our-health/pressure-ulcers-applying-all-our-health. (Accessed 10 Feb 2023).

Patel, H. W., Karamat, A., Saeed, M., Hassanein, M., Syed, A., Chowdhury, T. A., Farooqi, A., & Khunti, K. (2020). *The South Asian Health Foundation (UK) guidelines for managing diabetes during Ramadan: 2020 update* [pdf]. UK: The South Asian Health Foundation. Retrieved from https://static1.squarespace.com/static/5944e54ab3d2b94bb077ceb/t/5e847ebf2c6ec1680158c373/1585741505374/Ramadan+Guidelines+Update.pdf. Accessed 29 May 2022.

Patient Info. (2018). *Pressure sores.* Retrieved from https://patient.info/skin-conditions/pressure-sores. Accessed 26 May 2022.

RCN. (2021). *Debate: Male nurses.* Retrieved from https://www.rcn.org.uk/congress/congress-events/male-nurses. Accessed 29 May 2022.

Shi, C., Bonnett, L. J., Dumville, J. C., & Cullum, N. (2020). People with non-blanching erythema are at higher risk of pressure ulcers. *British Journal of Dermatology, 182*(2), e63. https://doi.org/10.1111/bjd.18154.

The Muslim Council of Britain. (2022). *Welcoming Ramadan 2022.* Retrieved from https://mcb.org.uk/resources/ramadan/. Accessed 26 May 2022.

Tonkin, T. (2019). *Senior doctor speaks out about racial abuse.* Retrieved from https://www.bma.org.uk/news-and-opinion/senior-doctor-speaks-out-about-racial-abuse. Accessed 26 May 2022.

Wound Source. (2017). *Tunnelling wound assessment and treatment.* Retrieved from https://www.woundsource.com/blog/tunneling-wound-assessment-and-treatment. Accessed 26 May 2022.

Wound Source. (2022a). *Pressure, stage 2.* Retrieved from https://www.woundsource.com/patientcondition/pressure-ulcers-stage-2. Accessed 26 May 2022.

Wound Source. (2022b). *Pressure, stage 3 and 4.* Retrieved from https://www.woundsource.com/patientcondition/pressure-ulcers-stages-3-and-4. Accessed 26 May 2022.

CHAPTER 24

End

I am now a qualified registered nurse and have been qualified for around 2 years and 4 months (as of May 2022). I started this journey off as a student nurse, wanting to get my head down and qualify then go back into sexual health as a sexual health nurse. My whole world changed as a student nurse, my ambitions changed, my sails were set, and then I qualified as a general practice (GP) nurse for 2 years, and my sails started to change direction. My passion started to turn into something a little different, that ambition turned into a new ambition and new goals, and I threw myself at every one of them head-on. I am now working on a number of different projects, such as delivering transgender healthcare webinars to healthcare settings as well as other settings, such as prison services along with providing help and information for people. I am now volunteering with a lesbian, gay, bisexual, and transgender (LGBT) charity and help run group sessions and their social media spaces. I am co-chair of the General Practice Nurse; Students and Nurses Network (GPNSNN) and am trying to make changes within primary care for students and newly qualified nurses. Please feel free to find us across social media platforms and get in contact if you need any help and advice on working in primary care. My next goal is to get into education and teach at university, I would love to be part of the future of nursing. Spoiler alert - I got into lecturing in December 2022 and I am getting married in April 2023! I have my happy ever after.

I have my own blog site and YouTube channel, and I am writing this book in the hope it will help at least one student nurse out there (if this is you reading this – thank you, it was all worth it to know I have hopefully, helped one person). I have no idea how my sails changed or how/why my ambitions changed during my journey, but I know that my journey is not over yet. With each step I take, a new idea, a new motivation and a new ambition in life is created.

So, my final piece of advice is, don't assume you know where life will take you, because you are going to be pleasantly surprised once you start your nursing career. Nursing has a huge world of opportunities if you just have the strength to go for it!

I don't know what the rest of my career holds, but I know that I have more ambition now than ever. My university and the people I have met on my journey have shaped me into the nurse I wanted to be, and I have achieved my goals and more. Even the bad times in my life that I have spoken about, I couldn't thank those people enough – the good, the bad and the ugly. I wouldn't go back and change a single thing. Because it has all led me to where I need to be today, and today shapes the way for my future, and I am excited and ready for it – whatever it brings.

So, despite not knowing what I wanted to be in life as a child, I finally found it and achieved my dream of becoming a nurse, and now I am putting my own stamp on the world.

And lastly, some motivational quotes and advice from other nursing professionals who I approached across social media for you.

Stay calm, the start of the course is very overwhelming. Just focus on the next placement and the next assignment. Don't look too far ahead. The knowledge and experience will take of itself I promise!

STUDENT NURSE FROM TWITTER

Schedule social time, time for yourself to do things you enjoy. Put it into their diaries, even if it means blocking out a section of time every week or day every so often but a minimum of 2 a month.

NURSE FROM TWITTER

Learn to prioritise. Sometimes assignments and placement will be the priority but sometimes YOU are the priority. Assignments can wait, but you need to be well to do well. So, take a break even if it's for a couple of days, remember your self-care, get some sleep and look after yourself.

LEARNING DISABILITY STUDENT NURSE FROM TWITTER

Always trust your instincts, enjoy the process of being a student nurse and you'll be amazed at how much you grow. It's how you change and evolve into a different person that keeps me going – all for the better and the excitement of almost being a registered nurse. Makes me proud and to show my daughters how strong we can be.

SECOND-YEAR STUDENT NURSE AND MOTHER

I was in my third year but struggling with placement, not sleeping well and was being quizzed over medications. I was told I couldn't use my notes, got a few wrong and because I relied on my notes, this meant 'you'll never be a nurse!' If that happens, prove them wrong!

UNIVERSITY LECTURER

Nursing is a vocation, we do it because we care. Always advocate for your patients and do the right thing. Never feel you cannot speak up, no matter what the medical area is.

NURSE

Nursing is what you do for a living, you can love it and you can be passionate about it. But they will replace you in a heartbeat once you're gone. Give your all to all aspects of life – not just the job.

GP NURSE CLINICAL MANAGER

Always do your best and good luck!
                                                    FIRST YEAR STUDENT NURSE

Don't compare yourself to others. I always worried that I had no previous care experience. I thought other students always seemed more confident and capable. I worried if they had mastered a skill that I hadn't tried yet! It is your journey, and you will find your own strengths.
                        REGISTERED NURSE AND LECTURER OF HEALTH SCIENCES

Comparison is the thief of joy, this is your journey, live it your way
                                                    MUM AND NURSE

Choose your first post-university job based on what you want and not what others think you should do. You'll save yourself a whole lot of trouble if you reach for the stars instead of something you don't enjoy.
                                        NEWLY QUALIFIED DISTRICT NURSE

Believe in yourself; have the confidence to ask; speak up and use your voice
                                                    DISTRICT NURSE (now retired)

You're not going to finish uni ready to be an experienced nurse like your mentors – but you will be ready to qualify at the end of the degree and the rest will come with time. Enjoy every second of being a student, because time really does fly by, and you will miss it once it's finished.
                                                    NEWLY QUALIFIED GP NURSE

Crying is alright in its way while it lasts. But you have to stop sooner or later and then you still have to decide what to do
                        CS LEWIS, THE SILVER CHAIR, CHRONICLES OF NARNIA

Despite what people say, you CAN go straight into primary care nursing!
                                                    GP NURSE

Find your people, those are the ones who will get you through
                                                    REGISTERED NURSE

Resilience and wellbeing are essential; you need to take care of you so you can care for others
                                                    DEPUTY CHIEF NURSE

The nurse who is the bully, put in a formal complaint about them. Don't put up with bad behaviour from anyone. What you tolerate will happen to others too
                                        REGISTERED MENTAL HEALTH NURSE

Everyone has their own journey so concentrate on yours
TWITTER NURSE

The only person you should try to be better than is the person you were the day before
REGISTERED NURSE

The only pressure you're feeling is the pressure you're putting on yourself
NURSE FROM TWITTER

Give and take nothing for granted
STUDENT NURSE

People will forget what you did, but people will never forget how you made them feel
MAYA ANGELOU

Nursing is about doing what you could and should have done. When you could and should have it.
NICK GEE (Associate Professor/Nurse)

The degree is hard, encourage every effort and keep your dream alive. A nurse doesn't de-skill, they re-skill wherever they choose to work.
STUDENT NURSE

When you feel down or face hardship, always remember why you started this course.
STUDENT PAEDIATRIC NURSE

You cannot pour from an empty cup. Take each day, step by step, day by day.
NURSING STUDENT AND BLOGGER

INDEX

Note: Page numbers followed by "*f*" indicate figures, "*t*" indicate tables, and "*b*" indicate boxes.